Metabolic Syndrome and Obesity in Childhood and Adolescence

Pediatric and Adolescent Medicine

Vol. 19

Series Editor

Wieland Kiess Leipzig

Metabolic Syndrome and Obesity in Childhood and Adolescence

Volume Editors

Wieland Kiess Leipzig
Martin Wabitsch Ulm
Claudio Maffeis Verona
Arya M. Sharma Edmonton, Alta.

28 figures, 18 in color, 9 tables, 2015

KARGER Basel · Freiburg · Paris · London · New York · Chennai · New Delhi · Bangkok · Beijing · Shanghai · Tokyo · Kuala Lumpur · Singapore · Sydney

Pediatric and Adolescent Medicine
Founded 1991 by D. Branski, Jerusalem

Prof. Wieland Kiess, MD
Department of Women and Child Health
Hospital for Children and Adolescents
University of Leipzig, Leipzig, Germany

Prof. Claudio Maffeis, MD
Pediatric Diabetes, Clinical Nutrition and Obesity
Department of Life and Reproduction Science
School of Medicine and Surgery
University of Verona, Verona, Italy

Prof. Martin Wabitsch, MD, PhD
Interdisciplinary Obesity Unit
Division of Pediatric Endocrinology and Diabetes
Department of Pediatrics and Adolescent Medicine
University Medical Center Ulm
University of Ulm, Ulm, Germany

Prof. Arya M. Sharma, MD, PhD, DSc. (h.c.), FRCPC
Obesity Research and Management
Division of Endocrinology
Department of Medicine
Faculty of Medicine and Dentistry
University of Alberta, Edmonton, Alta., Canada

Library of Congress Cataloging-in-Publication Data

Metabolic syndrome and obesity in childhood and adolescence /
volume editors, Wieland Kiess, Martin Wabitsch, Claudio Maffeis, Arya M. Sharma.
p. ; cm. -- (Pediatric and adolescent medicine, ISSN 1017-5989; vol. 19)
Includes bibliographical references and indexes.
ISBN 978-3-318-02798-3 (hard cover: alk. paper) -- ISBN 978-3-318-02799-0 (electronic version)
I. Kiess, W. (Wieland), editor. II. Wabitsch, Martin, editor. III. Maffeis, Claudio, editor.
IV. Sharma, Arya M., editor. V. Series: Pediatric and adolescent medicine; v. 19. 1017-5989
[DNLM: 1. Pediatric Obesity. 2. Adolescent. 3. Child. 4. Metabolic Syndrome X.
W1 PE163HL v. 19 2015 / WS 115]
RJ399.C6
618.92'39--dc23 2014044095

Bibliographic Indices. This publication is listed in bibliographic services, including Current Contents®.

Disclaimer. The statements, opinions and data contained in this publication are solely those of the individual authors and contributors and not of the publisher and the editor(s). The appearance of advertisements in the book is not a warranty, endorsement, or approval of the products or services advertised or of their effectiveness, quality or safety. The publisher and the editor(s) disclaim responsibility for any injury to persons or property resulting from any ideas, methods, instructions or products referred to in the content or advertisements.

Drug Dosage. The authors and the publisher have exerted every effort to ensure that drug selection and dosage set forth in this text are in accord with current recommendations and practice at the time of publication. However, in view of ongoing research, changes in government regulations, and the constant flow of information relating to drug therapy and drug reactions, the reader is urged to check the package insert for each drug for any change in indications and dosage and for added warnings and precautions. This is particularly important when the recommended agent is a new and/or infrequently employed drug.

www.karger.com
Printed in Germany on acid-free and non-aging paper (ISO 9706) by Kraft Druck GmbH, Ettlingen
ISSN 1017–5989
e-ISSN 1662–3886
ISBN 978–3–318–02798–3
e-ISBN 978–3–318–02799–0

KARGER 125 YEARS

Contents

Societal Aspects and Prevention

Obesity Management

Preface

In this volume in our series 'Pediatric and Adolescent Medicine,' probably the most common and most urgent clinical problem in pediatrics and adolescent medicine is being covered by experts from around the world. The volume discusses pertinent and prevalent topics such as the definition and clinical aspects of obesity. Additionally, novel viewpoints and ideas for the future are presented; these will facilitate both interaction with obese children and adolescents in a fair and appropriate way and collaboration with the individuals affected to seek appropriate and effective prevention and treatment measures.

In section number one, definitions and clinical aspects are covered. Martin Wabitsch from the University of Ulm, Germany, and Antje Körner from the University of Leipzig, Germany, discuss different definitions and the basic clinical aspects of obesity in childhood and adolescence. They describe obesity as part of metabolic syndrome and indeed as one of the causes leading to the full-blown clinical picture of metabolic syndrome. Abdullah Bereket from Istanbul, Turkey, and his co-workers report on the following in their chapter on the clinical entity of hypothalamic obesity: obesity caused by injury or trauma to or surgery on the hypothalamus as well as the fact that inborn genetic diseases affecting nuclei and regions of the hypothalamus can cause obesity in a very severe and extreme way. Abdullah Bereket and his colleagues emphasize that hypothalamic obesity is still resistant to traditional therapeutic measures, that prevention should be mandatory but is also difficult, and that new clinical trials with new treatment protocols are urgently required.

In section two, Yvonne Böttcher and Peter Kovacs from the University of Leipzig, Germany, first present a very nicely written chapter on the genetics of obesity in childhood and adolescence. They focus on DNA and methylation and the biology of the disease. Second, Hermann Kalhoff and Mathilde Kersting from Dortmund and Bonn, Germany, outline all aspects of nutrition in relation to metabolic syndrome and obesity in childhood and adolescence. Third, sedentary behavior has been identified as a public health issue for the last 10 years. This is being pointed out in the excellent chapter from France, in which Maïthé Tauber and her colleagues from Toulouse rightly argue that preventive interventions should focus on changing the sedentary lifestyle, even and especially at a young age. In this fine contribution they also report on why people adopt a sedentary lifestyle. Fourth, Sandra Plachta-Danielzik and Manfred James Müller from the University of Kiel, Germany, review their own data and perform a meta-analysis of all available information on socio-economic aspects as causes of metabolic syndrome and obesity. It is actually their contribution via the 'KOPS' study in Kiel that has drawn our attention to the socio-economic aspects of metabolic syndrome during the last decade.

In section three, the consequences of obesity in childhood and adolescence are discussed. Martin Wabitsch and Christian Denzer from the University of Ulm, Germany, review the impact of obesity on carbohydrate metabolism. They especially refer to insulin resistance, glucose intolerance, and the long-term development of type 2 diabetes early in life. Falk Thielemann, Klaus-Peter Guenther, and Maik Stiehler from the University of Dresden, Germany, discuss the orthopedic aspects of obesity in children and adults. In fact, back pain, hip and knee pain, and a vast array of orthopedic complications that are typical of severe obesity are already present in childhood. A very often neglected aspect of obesity at all ages, namely, urogenital complications, is summarized in the chapter by Anita Morandi and Claudio Maffeis from the University of Verona in Italy. In fact, renal disease, even including terminal renal failure as well as urolithiasis in the long term, and lower urinary tract symptoms such as itching, painful urination, and cystitis are already related to obesity in childhood and adolescence. The last chapter in this section deals with the putative consequences of obesity in childhood on pubertal development; it is still unclear whether obesity has led to an earlier onset of puberty in affected populations or whether the phenomena of the prevalence of obesity and an earlier age at menarche and puberty are merely coincidental. Our groups from the University of Leipzig in Germany and the University of Melbourne in Australia (authors Isabel V. Wagner, Matthew Sabin, and Wieland Kiess) summarize the available data.

In section four, the societal aspects and prevention of obesity are discussed. Indeed, during the last couple of years, it has become clear that societal aspects and indeed the social sciences have to be addressed much more when one wants to speak about obesity in childhood and adolescence. In fact, Ulrike Igel and Gesine Grande (University of Applied Sciences (HTWK), Leipzig, Germany) discuss the relationship between neighborhood characteristics and obesity in children and adolescents. This topic is very new, very pressing, and indeed innovative. Robert H. Lustig from the University of California, San Francisco, USA, writes about the role of food industries and the role of a 'Western' diet as causative factors in the development of obesity. He sets science and politics, as sometimes conflicting and sometimes counterproductive entities, as the focus of this chapter. Currently, the most talked about societal aspect in our lives seems to be economics; it is therefore understandable that an economic perspective on childhood obesity is also presented in this section. Rolf Holle and his colleagues from the University of Munich, Germany, do this in a very comprehensive, innovative, and diligent way. Finally, two chapters on new ways to think about prevention are presented by two young investigators from the University of Leipzig,

Germany. Jana Markert identifies barriers that are obstacles to families' participation in childhood obesity prevention programs. She draws from a large body of data that she and her co-workers have assembled and already partially published on this matter. Since electronic data usage and electronic communication means are now so prevalent in our lives, it is important to investigate e-health approaches and their effects on obesity prevention. Can electronic communication means and social networks be used for obesity prevention and even treatment (chapter by Sabine Herget, University of Leipzig)?

In section five, new obesity treatments are presented. Thomas Reinehr from Datteln, Germany, who has developed his own Obeldicks obesity treatment program and has successfully evaluated and institutionalized it, reviews available obesity programs, their efficacy, and their routine clinical use. Next, in one chapter, bariatric surgery in adolescents is reviewed: Paola Luca, Elizabeth Dettmer, Jakob C. Langer, and Jill K. Hamilton from Calgary and Toronto, Canada, report on the current status of adolescent bariatric surgery as an evolving field. Lastly, Geoff D.C. Ball and co-workers from several Canadian Universities describe their vast experience and insights related to working effectively with families and operating within the health-care system to manage pediatric obesity. It is important that in this last contribution in our volume, Geoff D.C. Ball and co-authors in fact go far beyond mere 'weight loss' and describe the many aspects of metabolic syndrome and obesity in childhood and adolescence once more in a comprehensive and interdisciplinary manner.

Wieland Kiess, Leipzig
Martin Wabitsch, Ulm
Claudio Maffeis, Verona
Arya M. Sharma, Edmonton, Alta.

Kiess W, Wabitsch M, Maffeis C, Sharma AM (eds): Metabolic Syndrome and Obesity in Childhood and Adolescence.
Pediatr Adolesc Med. Basel, Karger, 2015, vol 19, pp 1–12 (DOI: 10.1159/000368101)

Definitions

Martin Wabitsch[a] · Antje Körner[b]

[a]Interdisciplinary Obesity Unit, Division of Pediatric Endocrinology and Diabetes, Department of Pediatrics and Adolescent Medicine, University Medical Center Ulm, University of Ulm, Ulm, and [b]IFB AdiposityDiseases, Medical Faculty, University of Leipzig, Leipzig, Germany

Abstract

It has long been recognized that some classical risk factors for cardiovascular disease occur in clusters. This combined presence of several risk factors has been termed metabolic syndrome. Nevertheless, the selection and definition of these risk factors with cut-off values is not without controversy. Particularly in children, the definition of metabolic syndrome is even more complicated, not only because children present with early stages of metabolic and cardiovascular alterations but also due to aspects of physical and pubertal development; thus, age-corrected cut-off values need to be regarded.

Introduction

The co-occurrence of the risk factors of (visceral) obesity, hypertension, dyslipidemia, insulin resistance and possibly disturbed glucose regulation in an individual is associated with significantly increased risks of cardiovascular disease and type 2 diabetes mellitus that contribute to increased mortality. Longitudinal studies have shown that the presence of these risk factors during childhood and adolescence leads to early-onset arteriosclerosis. The clinical manifestation of arteriosclerosis is usually only recognized at the advanced stage because clinical symptoms typically only include marked stenosis (>70%) of the coronary arteries or of the cerebral (or leg) arteries. However, long before the manifestation of arteriosclerosis is clinically evident, there are frequently subclinical alterations of vessels that occur over many years and manifest as endothelial dysfunction, fatty streaks, the swelling of the intima and media and plaques. This fact has been markedly demonstrated by autopsy studies (e.g. the PDAY study), which have shown the first fatty streaks in normal, healthy, young individuals who died as a result of an accident or homicide during the second decade of life. The occurrence and extent of these atherosclerotic lesions are significantly increased in overweight or obese individuals.

It is well recognized that several risk factors occur more often together and can cause diseases like myocardial infarction and stroke. Nevertheless, the term metabolic syndrome (MetS) has found its way into clinical medicine only in the last years and has recently been established in pediatric and adolescent medicine [1, 2].

In the 1950s, Jean Vague [3] recognized that the co-occurrence of obesity with abdominal body fat distribution, hypertension, diabetes and hyperuricemia leads to arteriosclerosis. In 1988, the American diabetologist Gerald M. Reaven [4] described the so-called syndrome X, which is a complex syndrome consisting of insulin resistance, hyperinsulinemia, hypertriglyceridemia, reduced high-density lipoprotein (HDL) cholesterol, hypertension and disturbed glucose tolerance. Finally, Kaplan [5] spoke memorably of a 'deadly quartet' consisting of abdominal obesity, hypertension, impaired glucose tolerance and hypertriglyceridemia. Considering that the first sequelae of obesity that are part of the above-mentioned complex already occur during childhood and that the first vascular alterations are detectable during early adulthood, the existence of this complete symptom complex during childhood is likely. MetS was characterized in 1991 in pediatric and adolescent medicine and was examined and discussed afterwards by physicians of national and international pediatric societies [6]. Nevertheless, definitions in pediatric populations are more complicated due to the age range that has to be covered and the limitations in the normal cut-off and reference values.

Definitions

The symptom complex consisting of obesity with abdominal body fat distribution, dyslipidemia (hypertriglyceridemia and reduced HDL cholesterol), insulin resistance and impaired glucose tolerance as well as arterial hypertension is known in adults as MetS.

The corresponding symptoms occur in individuals in combinations ('clustering') more often than what would be expected by mere coincidence. A similar constellation of risk factors has been found in obese children.

Additional typical findings associated with MetS that can occur during adolescence are non-alcoholic fatty liver disease, hyperuricemia, polycystic ovarian syndrome and microalbuminuria.

Interestingly, a clustering of cardiovascular risk factors has also been often observed in family members. In the parental and grandparental generations, secondary complications or endpoints (early-onset myocardial infarction and stroke) are frequently present. This information about family history is important for the assessment of the health risk of the affected child or adolescent, even though it is not an official criterion for pediatric MetS.

The term 'tracking', which is often used in relation to MetS, means the persistence of individual risk factors from childhood to adulthood as well as the increasing expression of the risk factors with age. These correlations can be interpreted as follows: if evidence of MetS is found in a patient, symptoms will quite likely persist to later in life, and individual clinical symptoms will develop with age. Nevertheless, physiological variations in some parameters during development need to be considered. For example, during pubertal development, transient insulin resistance is also present in healthy lean children, even though the magnitude of this alteration is much lower compared to obesity-related insulin resistance.

There is currently no generally accepted definition of MetS during childhood and adolescence with indications for limit values for the individual components. The aim to develop a definition for child and adolescent MetS with a preferably high clinical relevance is barely accessible at the moment because this syndrome describes a health risk, and there are no sufficient long term data on clinical endpoints that allow for the determination of individual reference values and their combinations to delineate a prognostic risk. In addition, in children and adolescents, it is not possible to indicate reference values for the individual components of MetS based on development because the presence of these components depends on age and puberty.

In 2007, the International Diabetes Federation [7] proposed a definition of MetS in children and adolescents, which is shown in table 1a, b. This rather conservative definition is well applicable in practice and takes into account developmental aspects (tracking). Until better definitions of MetS are available, the International Diabetes Federation definition of this syndrome for children and adolescents is proposed for use in practice.

The assessment of cardiovascular risk in children and adolescents in relation to the presence of MetS and possibly the indication of an effective therapy should be stratified independent of an exact definition of this syndrome.

Reference Values for the Individual Components of Metabolic Syndrome

The German Working Group of Obesity in Children and Adolescents guidelines [8] recommend the use of the following reference values for the diagnostic assessment of cardiovascular risk factors, which are conjunct in MetS.

Visceral Obesity

In accordance with several national and international guidelines, obesity is defined by the reference values for body mass index (BMI), even though distinct cut offs exist for the definition of overweight and obesity in different countries ranging from the 80th to the 97th percentile [9].

An assessment of abdominal fat distribution can be made by measuring waist circumference. For this, the patient should be lightly dressed (in underwear), upright, and standing in straight view with their arms hanging at the side of the body and the body weight evenly distributed on both legs. The patient should inhale and exhale quietly. For the measurement (measuring accuracy of +/– 1 mm), a non-elastic measuring tape is applied to the area of the strongest medial indentation of the body side

Table 1. Consensus definition of metabolic syndrome in children and adolescents as reported by the International Diabetes Federation

a Age groups

Age 6 to <10 years
Obesity is defined as a waist circumference of >90th percentile.
MetS cannot be diagnosed, but further measurements should be made if there is a family history of MetS, type 2 diabetes mellitus, dyslipidemia, cardiovascular disease, hypertension, or obesity.
The IDF suggests that a strong message for weight reduction should be delivered to patients with abdominal obesity.

Age 10 to <16 years
Obesity is defined as a waist circumference of >90th percentile (or adult cut-off if lower).
Triglycerides >1.7 mmol/l
HDL cholesterol <1.03 mmol/l
BP >130 mmHg systolic or 85 mmHg diastolic
Glucose >5.6 mmol/l (oral glucose tolerance test recommended) or known type 2 diabetes mellitus

Age >16 years
Use existing IDF criteria for adults. According to the new IDF definition, for a person to be defined as having MetS, they must have central obesity (defined as waist circumference[a] using ethnicity-specific values) plus any two of the following four factors:

- raised triglyceride levels: >150 mg/dl (1.7 mmol/l) or specific treatment for this lipid abnormality
- reduced HDL cholesterol: <40 mg/dl (1.03 mmol/l) in males and <50 mg/dl (1.29 mmol/l) in females, or specific treatment for this lipid abnormality and the following:
- raised BP: SBP of >130 mmHg or DBP of 85 mmHg or treatment of previously diagnosed hypertension
- raised fasting plasma glucose: >100 mg/dl (5.6 mmol/l) or previously diagnosed type 2 diabetes (if above 5.6 mmol/l or 100 mg/dl, the oral glucose tolerance test is strongly recommended but is not necessary to define the presence of this syndrome).

b Waist circumference by origin

Country/ethnic group	Sex	Waist circumference, cm
Europids[b]	Male	>94
	Female	>80
South Asians[c]	Male	>90
	Female	>80
Chinese	Male	>90
	Female	>80
Japanese[d]	Male	>90
	Female	>80
Ethnic South and Central Americans	Use South Asian recommendations until more specific data are available	
Sub-Saharan Africans	Use European data until more specific data are available	
Eastern Mediterranean and Middle East (Arab) populations	Use European data until more specific data are available	

Table 1. Continued

Children younger than 6 years of age were excluded from the definition because of insufficient data for this age group.
[a] If BMI is >30, central obesity can be assumed, and waist circumference does not need to be measured.
[b] In the USA, ATP III values (102 cm for males, and 88 cm for females) are likely to be continued to be used for clinical purposes In future epidemiological studies of populations of Europid origin. Prevalence should be determined using both European and North American cut-off points to allow for better comparisons.
[c] Based on a population of Chinese, Malay and Asian-Indian individuals.
[d] Subsequent data analyses have suggested that the Asian values (90 cm for males, and 80 cm for females) should be used for Japanese populations until more data are available.
IDF = International Diabetes Foundation; SBP = systolic blood pressure; DBP = diastolic blood pressure.

structure between the lower costal arch and the iliac crest. If an indentation in the waist region is not recognizable, the waist circumference should be measured between the iliac crest and costal arch. The measuring tape is applied horizontally to the ground and under tension (not denting the abdominal wall), and the measured value is read after expiration by the patient. To minimize errors, the measurement should be repeated, and the mean value should be calculated from the two measurements.

Waist circumference is also subject to age- and gender/sex-specific alterations. In 2008, Kromeyer-Hauschild et al. [10] published age- and gender-specific percentiles for the waist circumferences of 6- to 18-year-old German children and adolescents (fig. 1a, b) [10]. In adults, abdominal obesity is defined by waist circumferences of ≥80 (female) and ≥94 cm (male) [11]. In contrast, there is no uniform limit value reported in the literature for children and adolescents. Waist circumference and BMI correlate at a high level [10]. To identify increased abdominal fat accumulation in children and adolescents, a waist circumference of above the 90th percentile is the recommended criterion based on the definition of obesity in these age groups (BMI >90th percentile).

In addition to the waist circumference, waist-to-hip ratio and more recently, waist-to-height, are parameters for assessing fat distribution. The latter is supposed to have the advantage of being more age independent, and a uniform cut-off of 0.5 could be applied. However, it is not considered a criterion for the official MetS definition.

Dyslipidemia

The determination of fasting lipid levels (total cholesterol; low-density lipoprotein, HDL, and triglycerides) is part of the basic diagnosis for all obese children and adolescents as well as overweight children and adolescents with risk factors, e.g. a positive family history of early cardiovascular disease. Reference values are available for the diagnostic evaluation of lipid levels (table 2).

Values beyond the target range should be followed. The assessment of altered lipid values can only occur by taking into account all cardiovascular risk factors. Any necessary dietary or pharmacological interventions should be made in accordance with the guidelines of the American Academy of Pediatrics.

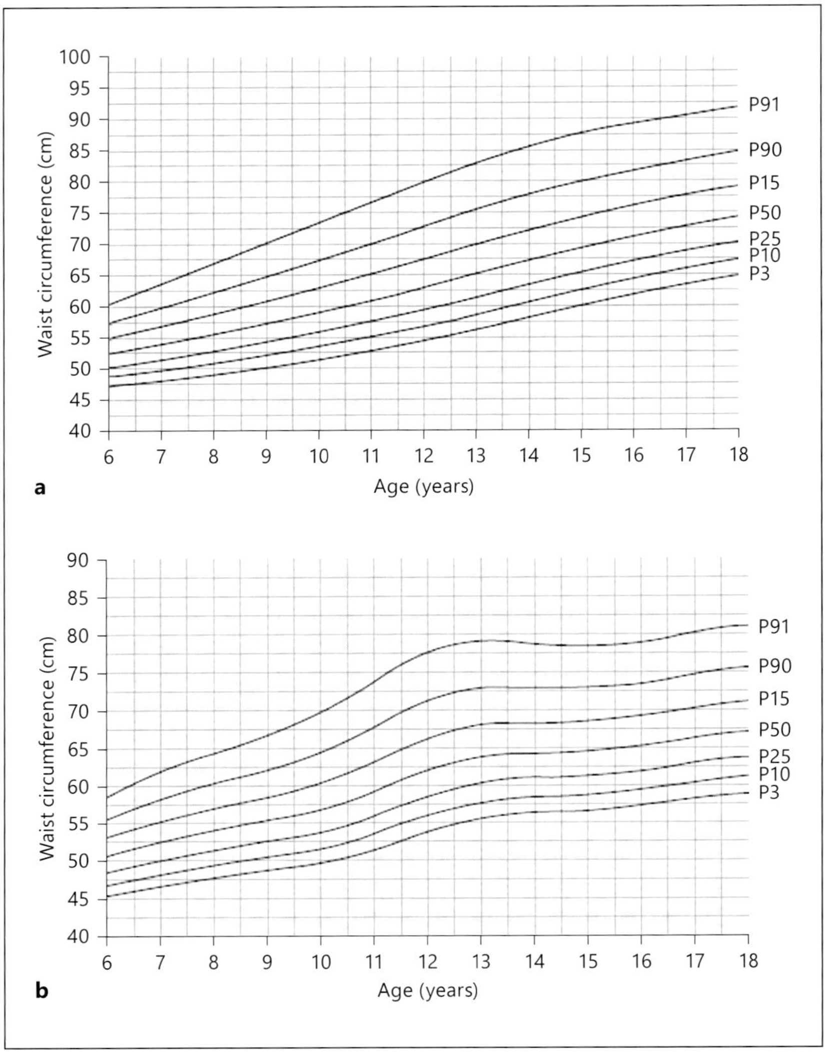

Fig. 1. a Percentile graph of waist circumferences (boys 6–18 years) by Kromeyer-Hauschild et al. (2008). **b** Percentile graph of waist circumferences (girls 6–18 years) by Kromeyer-Hauschild et al. (2008).

Arterial Hypertension

Blood pressure (BP) should be measured with the patient in an upright sitting position using the right arm in a quiet environment after a 5-minute period of rest. The use of the right cuff width (to cover at least 80% of the upper arm length) is important. The measured values must be interpreted on the basis of sex-, age- and body height-specific reference values (for an example of the reference values, see table 3a, b). The classification of hypertension in children and adolescents with measurement frequencies and therapy recommendations is shown in table 4.

Table 2. Acceptable, borderline-high, and high plasma lipid, lipoprotein, and apolipoprotein concentrations for children and adolescents according to the American Academy of Pediatrics (see www.aap.org)

Category	Low, mg/dl[a]	Acceptable, mg/dl	Borderline-High, mg/dl	High, mg/dl[a]
Total cholesterol	–	<170	170–199	≥200
LDL cholesterol	–	<110	110–129	≥130
Non-HDL cholesterol	–	<120	120–144	≥145
Apolipoprotein B	–	<90	90–109	≥110
Triglycerides				
0–9 years	–	<75	75–99	≥100
10–19 years	–	<90	90–129	≥130
HDL cholesterol	<40	>45	40–45	–
Apolipoprotein A-1	<115	>120	115–120	–

[a] The low cut-off points for HDL cholesterol and apolipoprotein A-1 represent approximately the 10th percentile. The cut-off points for high and borderline-high represent approximately the 95th and 75th percentiles, respectively. LDL = low-density lipoprotein.

With unclear or marginal results and to confirm the diagnosis of arterial hypertension, an ambulatory 24-hour BP measurement should be performed. The assessment of the 24-hour BP measurement is also based on appropriate reference values [12, 13].

Insulin Resistance and Glucose Regulation Disorder

A frequent clinical sign indicating hyperinsulinemia is acanthosis nigricans, which is a dirty-brownish hyperpigmentation of the skin with a coarsening of its appearance, which occurs typically in the neck and armpits (fig. 2).

The determination of the fasting serum insulin concentration allows for the calculation of insulin resistance indices (e.g. homeostasis model assessment of insulin resistance or quantitative insulin sensitivity check index). However, because of the high intraindividual variability of these indices, verifying their significance is a challenge. It must also be considered that methodologies of glucose and insulin determination have not yet been standardized. The gold standard for the measurement of insulin resistance is the euglycemic hyperinsulinemia clamp, which is a time consuming, invasive and expensive method that is only suitable for scientific questioning. A more clinically applicable test is the oral glucose tolerance test, which is performed following the guidelines of the American Diabetes Association [14]. An oral dose of liquid glucose (1 g glucose/kg body weight, max. 75 g) is given to the patient, and the blood glucose response is measured. Unfortunately, current guidelines provide reference ranges only for fasting levels of glucose and insulin and for 120-minute glucose levels (table 5). Also, oral glucose tolerance test results have shown high intra-individual variability. This is in part due to the arbitrary 120-minute time point of glucose

Table 3. Standard values for single random blood pressure measurement according to the American Academy of Pediatrics (see www.aap.org)

a Boys

Age, years	BP percentile	Percentile of height													
		SBP, mmHg							DBP, mmHg						
		5th	10th	25th	50th	75th	90th	95th	5th	10th	25th	50th	75th	90th	95th
6	50th	91	92	94	96	98	99	100	53	53	54	55	56	57	57
	90th	105	106	108	110	111	113	113	68	68	69	70	71	72	72
	95th	109	110	112	114	115	117	117	72	72	73	74	75	76	76
	99th	116	117	119	121	123	124	125	80	80	81	82	83	84	84
7	50th	92	94	95	97	99	100	101	55	55	56	57	58	59	59
	90th	106	107	109	111	113	114	115	70	70	71	72	73	74	74
	95th	110	111	113	115	117	118	119	74	74	75	76	77	78	78
	99th	117	118	120	122	124	125	126	82	82	83	84	85	86	86
8	50th	94	95	97	99	100	102	102	56	57	58	59	60	60	61
	90th	107	109	110	112	114	115	116	71	72	72	73	74	75	76
	95th	111	112	114	116	118	119	120	75	76	77	78	79	79	80
	99th	119	120	122	123	125	127	127	83	84	85	86	87	87	88
9	50th	95	96	98	100	102	103	104	57	58	59	60	61	61	62
	90th	109	110	112	114	115	117	118	72	73	74	75	76	76	77
	95th	113	114	116	118	119	121	121	76	77	78	79	80	81	81
	99th	120	121	123	125	127	128	129	84	85	86	87	88	88	89
10	50th	97	98	100	102	103	105	106	58	59	60	61	61	62	63
	90th	111	112	114	115	117	119	119	73	73	74	75	76	77	78
	95th	115	116	117	119	121	122	123	77	78	79	80	81	81	82
	99th	122	123	125	127	128	130	130	85	86	86	88	88	89	90
11	50th	99	100	102	104	105	107	107	59	59	60	61	62	63	63
	90th	113	114	115	117	119	120	121	74	74	75	76	77	78	78
	95th	117	118	119	121	123	124	125	78	78	79	80	81	82	82
	99th	124	125	127	129	130	132	132	86	86	87	88	89	90	90
12	50th	101	102	104	106	108	109	110	59	60	61	62	63	63	64
	90th	115	116	118	120	121	123	123	74	75	75	76	77	78	79
	95th	119	120	122	123	125	127	127	78	79	80	81	82	82	83
	99th	126	127	129	131	133	134	135	86	87	88	89	90	90	91
13	50th	104	105	106	108	110	111	112	60	60	61	62	63	64	64
	90th	117	118	120	122	124	125	126	75	75	76	77	78	79	79
	95th	121	122	124	126	128	129	130	79	79	80	81	82	83	83
	99th	128	130	131	133	135	136	137	87	87	88	89	90	91	91
14	50th	106	107	109	111	113	114	115	60	61	62	63	64	65	65
	90th	120	121	123	125	126	128	128	75	76	77	78	79	79	80
	95th	124	125	127	128	130	132	132	80	80	81	82	83	84	84
	99th	131	132	134	136	138	139	140	87	88	89	90	91	92	92
15	50th	109	110	112	113	115	117	117	61	62	63	64	65	66	66
	90th	122	124	125	127	129	130	131	76	77	78	79	80	80	81
	95th	126	127	129	131	133	134	135	81	81	82	83	84	85	85
	99th	134	135	136	138	140	142	142	88	89	90	91	92	93	93
16	50th	111	112	114	116	118	119	120	63	63	64	65	66	67	67
	90th	125	126	128	130	131	133	134	78	78	79	80	81	82	82
	95th	129	130	132	134	135	137	137	82	83	83	84	85	86	87
	99th	136	137	139	141	143	144	145	90	90	91	92	93	94	94
17	50th	114	115	116	118	120	121	122	65	66	66	67	68	69	70
	90th	127	128	130	132	134	135	136	80	80	81	82	83	84	84
	95th	131	132	134	136	138	139	140	84	85	86	87	87	88	89
	99th	139	140	141	143	145	146	147	92	93	93	94	95	96	97

Table 3. Continued

b Girls

Age, years	BP percentile	Percentile of height SBP, mmHg							Percentile of height DBP, mmHg						
		5th	10th	25th	50th	75th	90th	95th	5th	10th	25th	50th	75th	90th	95th
6	50th	91	92	93	94	96	97	98	54	54	55	56	56	57	58
	90th	104	105	106	108	109	110	111	68	68	69	70	70	71	72
	95th	108	109	110	111	113	114	115	72	72	73	74	74	75	76
	99th	115	116	117	119	120	121	122	80	80	80	81	82	83	83
7	50th	93	93	95	96	97	99	99	55	56	56	57	58	58	59
	90th	106	107	108	109	111	112	113	69	70	70	71	72	72	73
	95th	110	111	112	113	115	116	116	73	74	74	75	76	76	77
	99th	117	118	119	120	122	123	124	81	81	82	82	83	84	84
8	50th	95	95	96	98	99	100	101	57	57	57	58	59	60	60
	90th	108	109	110	111	113	114	114	71	71	71	72	73	74	74
	95th	112	112	114	115	116	118	118	75	75	75	76	77	78	78
	99th	119	120	121	122	123	125	125	82	82	83	83	84	85	86
9	50th	96	97	98	100	101	102	103	58	58	58	59	60	61	61
	90th	110	110	112	113	114	116	116	72	72	72	73	74	75	75
	95th	114	114	115	117	118	119	120	76	76	76	77	78	79	79
	99th	121	121	123	124	125	127	127	83	83	84	84	85	86	87
10	50th	98	99	100	102	103	104	105	59	59	59	60	61	62	62
	90th	112	112	114	115	116	118	118	73	73	73	74	75	76	76
	95th	116	116	117	119	120	121	122	77	77	77	78	79	80	80
	99th	123	123	125	126	127	129	129	84	84	85	86	86	87	88
11	50th	100	101	102	103	105	106	107	60	60	60	61	62	63	63
	90th	114	114	116	117	118	119	120	74	74	74	75	76	77	77
	95th	118	118	119	121	122	123	124	78	78	78	79	80	81	81
	99th	125	125	126	128	129	130	131	85	85	86	87	87	88	89
12	50th	102	103	104	105	107	108	109	61	61	61	62	63	64	64
	90th	116	116	117	119	120	121	122	75	75	75	76	77	78	78
	95th	119	120	121	123	124	125	126	79	79	79	80	81	82	82
	99th	127	127	128	130	131	132	133	86	86	87	88	88	89	90
13	50th	104	105	106	107	109	110	110	62	62	62	63	64	65	65
	90th	117	118	119	121	122	123	124	76	76	76	77	78	79	79
	95th	121	122	123	124	126	127	128	80	80	80	81	82	83	83
	99th	128	129	130	132	133	134	135	87	87	88	89	89	90	91
14	50th	106	106	107	109	110	111	112	63	63	63	64	65	66	66
	90th	119	120	121	122	124	125	125	77	77	77	78	79	80	80
	95th	123	123	125	126	127	129	129	81	81	81	82	83	84	84
	99th	130	131	132	133	135	136	136	88	88	89	90	90	91	92
15	50th	107	108	109	110	111	113	113	64	64	64	65	66	67	67
	90th	120	121	122	123	125	126	127	78	78	78	79	80	81	81
	95th	124	125	126	127	129	130	131	82	82	82	83	84	85	85
	99th	131	132	133	134	136	137	138	89	89	90	91	91	92	93
16	50th	108	108	110	111	112	114	114	64	64	65	66	66	67	68
	90th	121	122	123	124	126	127	128	78	78	79	80	81	81	82
	95th	125	126	127	128	130	131	132	82	82	83	84	85	85	86
	99th	132	133	134	135	137	138	139	90	90	90	91	92	93	93
17	50th	108	109	110	111	113	114	115	64	65	65	66	67	67	68
	90th	122	122	123	125	126	127	128	78	79	79	80	81	81	82
	95th	125	126	127	129	130	131	132	82	83	83	84	85	85	86
	99th	133	133	134	136	137	138	139	90	90	91	91	92	93	93

* The 90th percentile is 1.28 SD, the 95th percentile is 1.645 SD, and the 99th percentile is 2.326 SD over the mean.

Table 4. Classification of hypertension in children and adolescents, with measurement frequencies and therapy recommendations

	SBP or DBP percentile*	Frequency of BP measurement	Therapeutic lifestyle changes	Pharmacologic therapy
Normal	<90th	Recheck at next scheduled physical examination	Encourage healthy diet, sleep, and physical activity	–
Pre-hypertension	90th to <95th or if BP exceeds 120/80, or even if BP <90th percentile up to <95th percentile†	Recheck in 6 months	Weight-management counseling if overweight, and introduction of physical activity and diet management‡	None unless compelling indications are present, such as chronic kidney disease, diabetes mellitus, heart failure, or LVH exist
Stage 1 hypertension	95th to 99th percentile plus 5 mmHg	Recheck in 1–2 weeks or sooner if the patient is symptomatic; if persistently elevated on 2 additional occasions, evaluate or refer to source of care within 1 month	Weight-management counseling if overweight, and introduction of physical activity and diet management‡	Initiate therapy if hypertension persists despite a trial of four to six months of nonpharmacologic therapy or if compelling indications (as shown above) exist
Stage 2 hypertension	>99th percentile plus 5 mmHg	Evaluate or refer to source of care within 1 week or immediately if the patient is symptomatic	Weight-management counseling if overweight, and introduction of physical activity and diet management‡	Initiate therapy§

* For gender, age, and height measured on at least 3 separate occasions, if the systolic and diastolic categories are different, categorize by the higher value.
† This occurs typically at 12 years old for SBP and at 16 years old for DBP.
‡ Parents and children trying to modify their eating plans according to the Dietary Approaches to Stop Hypertension Study could benefit from consultation with a registered or licensed nutritionist to get them started.
§ More than 1 drug may be required.
LVH = left ventricular hypertrophy.

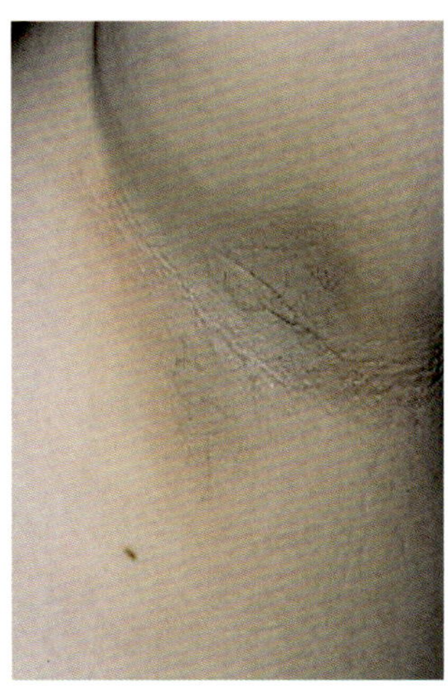

Fig. 2. Typical appearance of the axillary skin in a patient with acanthosis nigricans.

Table 5. Cut-off values for glucose and HbA1C

Parameter	HbA1C, %	FPG	2h PG oGTT
Diabetes	>6.5	>7.0 mmol/l >126 mg/dl	>11.0 mmol/l >200 mg/dl
Impaired glucose tolerance	5.7–6.4	5.6–6.9 mmol/l 100–125 mg/dl	7.8–11.0 mmol/l 140–199 mg/dl
Normal	≤5.7	≤5.6 mmol/l ≤99 mg/dl	≤7.8 mmol/l ≤139 mg/dl

FPG = fasting plasma glucose; 2h PG oGTT = plasma glucose at 120 min after ingestion of 1 g/kg (max 75 g) glucose.

measurement, which disregards the dynamic response of the glucose and insulin course.

This test also does not consider the insulin response and hence cannot detect hyperinsulinemia, which is the first sign of impaired glucose-insulin metabolism. More reference values for insulin, preferably in relation to the glucose response, are desirable.

The recommendation of the American Diabetes Association should be applied to children and adolescents beginning at age 10 or at the onset of puberty (whichever comes first) to 19 years of age to screen for type 2 diabetes (see www.diabetes.org).

Acknowledgements

The author thanks Bettina Wabitsch for her expert secretarial assistance. This chapter was written on the basis of an article in the *Journal of the Germany Society for Pediatrics and Adolescent Medicine* [15].

References

1 Denzer C, Wabitsch M: Das MetS bei Kindern und Jugendlichen; in Wirth A (ed) Das Metabolische Syndrom: München, Urban & Vogel, 2007, pp 30–41.

2 Wiegand S, l'Allemand D, Holl R, et al: Das Metabolische Syndrom bei Kindern und Jugendlichen: Konsensbasierte Leitlinie zur Diagnostik, Therapie und Prävention der Adipositas im Kindes- und Jugendalter. AGA, Berlin, 2011, http://www.a-g-a.de (accessed November 29, 2011).

3 Vague J: The degree of masculine differentiation of obesities: a factor determining predisposition to diabetes, atherosclerosis, gout, and uric calculous disease. Am J Clin Nutr 1956;4:20–34.

4 Reaven GM: Banting lecture 1988. Role of insulin resistance in human disease. Diabetes 1988;37:1595–1607.

5 Kaplan NM: The deadly quartet. Upper-body obesity, glucose intolerance, hypertriglyceridemia, and hypertension. Arch Intern Med 1989;149:1514–1520.

6 Wabitsch M, Hauner H, Heinze E, et al: The relationship between body fat distribution, fasting insulin levels and blood pressure in 79 obese adolescent girls. Abstracts 30th Annual Meeting European Society for Pediatric Endocrinology, Berlin, 1991.
7 International Diabetes Federation: The IDF Consensus Definition of the Metabolic Syndrome in Children and Adolescents. Brussels, IDF Communications, 2007.
8 Wabitsch M, Kunze D: Konsensbasierte Leitlinie zur Diagnostik, Therapie und Prävention der Adipositas im Kindes- und Jugendalter. 2013. www.a-g-a.de (accessed November 15, 2014).
9 Arbeitsgemeinschaft Adipositas im Kindes- und Jugendalter, Wabitsch M, Moss A, et al: Evidenzbasierte Leitlinie Therapie der Adipositas im Kindes- und Jugendalter (S3-Leitlinie). 2009. http://www.a-g-a.de (accessed November 29, 2011).
10 Kromeyer-Hauschild K, Glässer N, Zellner K: Perzentile für den Taillenumfang von Jenaer Kindern im Alter von 6 bis 18 Jahren. Aktuel Ernahrungsmed 2008;33:116–122.
11 Alberti K, Zimmet P, Shaw J, et al: IDF Epidemiological Task Force Consensus Group: The metabolic syndrome – a new worldwide definition. Lancet 2005;366:1059–1062.
12 Soergel M, Kirschstein M, Busch C, et al: Oscillometric twenty-four-hour ambulatory blood pressure values in healthy children and adolescents: a multicenter trial including 1141 subjects. J Pediatr 1997; 130:178–184.
13 Wühl E, Witte K, Soergel M, et al: Distribution of 24-h ambulatory blood pressure in children: normalized reference values and role of body dimensions. J Hypertens 2002;20:1995–2007.
14 American Diabetes Association: Standards of medical care in diabetes–2014. Diabetes Care 2014; 37(Suppl 1):S14–S80.
15 Wabitsch M, Moss A, Denzer C, et al: Das metabolische Syndrom. Monatsschr Kinderheilkd 2012;160: 277–292.

Martin Wabitsch, MD, PhD
Interdisciplinary Obesity Unit, Division of Pediatric Endocrinology and Diabetes
Department of Pediatrics and Adolescent Medicine
University Medical Center Ulm, University of Ulm
Eythstrasse 24, DE–89075 Ulm (Germany)
E-Mail martin.wabitsch@uniklinik-ulm.de

Kiess W, Wabitsch M, Maffeis C, Sharma AM (eds): Metabolic Syndrome and Obesity in Childhood and Adolescence.
Pediatr Adolesc Med. Basel, Karger, 2015, vol 19, pp 13–30 (DOI: 10.1159/000368102)

Hypothalamic Obesity in Children

Abdullah Bereket[a] · Wieland Kiess[c] · Robert H. Lustig[e] · Hermann L. Muller[d] · Anthony P. Goldstone[f] · Ram Weiss[g] · Yunus Yavuz[b] · Ze'ev Hochberg[h]

[a]Department of Paediatrics, Marmara University, Istanbul, and [b]Centre for Bariatric Surgery, Bilim University, Istanbul, Turkey; [c]Department of Women and Child Health, Hospital for Children and Adolescents, University of Leipzig, Leipzig, and [d]Department of Pediatrics, Klinikum Oldenburg, Oldenburg, Germany; [e]Department of Pediatrics, University of California, San Francisco, Calif., USA; [f]Metabolic and Molecular Imaging Group, MRC Clinical Sciences Centre, Imperial College London, Hammersmith Hospital, London, UK; [g]Department of Human Nutrition and Metabolism, Hebrew University School of Medicine, Jerusalem, and [h]Rambam Medical Centre and Rappaport Family Faculty of Medicine and Research Institute, Technion – Israel Institute of Technology, Haifa, Israel

Abstract

Hypothalamic obesity (HyOb) is a severe and rapidly developing form of obesity that was initially described in patients with hypothalamic tumours and surgical damage. However, this definition has now expanded to include obesity developing after a variety of insults to hypothalamic centres, such as infections, infiltrations, trauma, vascular problems, and hydrocephalus in addition to acquired or congenital functional defects in central energy homeostasis. The pathogenetic mechanisms underlying HyOb are complex and multifactorial. Weight gain results from damage to the ventromedial hypothalamus, which may lead to hyperphagia, a low resting metabolic rate, autonomic imbalance, growth hormone, gonadotropin and thyroid-stimulating hormone deficiencies, hypomobility and insomnia. Disruption of leptin signalling and decreased central sympathetic output seem to have a critical role in the development of HyOb. Surgical strategies to preserve hypothalamic integrity are mandatory for the prevention of HyOb in patients with craniopharyngioma or other hypothalamic tumours. At present, there is no standard pharmacological intervention that has been shown to consistently help these complicated patients. In select cases, octreotide seems to be effective when introduced early after the cranial insult. The safety and effectiveness of bariatric surgery in the management of HyOb has also not been well established. A general overview on HyOb with special emphasis on craniopharyngioma and Prader-Willi syndrome is provided in this chapter.

Introduction

The concept of hypothalamic obesity (HyOb) was first described in the early 20th century when two case reports of hypothalamic tumours producing obesity were published [1, 2]. Since then, this term has evolved first into obesity following surgery for

Table 1. Aetiologies of HyOb

Tumours: Craniopharyngioma, angiosarcoma, cholesteatoma, chordoma, colloid cysts, endothelioma, ependymoma, epidermoid, epithelioma, ganglioneuroma, germinoma, glioma, hamartoma, Langerhans cell, leukaemia, meningioma, pituitary macroadenoma, pinealoma, teratoma, metastases
Inflammatory: sarcoidosis, tuberculosis, arachnoiditis, histiocytosis X, encephalitis
Head trauma
Neurosurgery
Cranial radiotherapy
Cerebral aneurysm
Single gene mutations: Leptin, leptin receptor, CART, POMC, prohormone convertase-1, MC4R, BDNF (TrkB), single-minded 1 (Sim-1)
Genetic syndromes: Prader-Willi syndrome, Bardet-Biedl syndrome
Rapid-onset obesity with hypothalamic dysfunction, hypoventilation, and autonomic dysregulation (ROHHAD) syndrome
Psychotropic drugs: Antidepressants, mood stabilisers, antipsychotics

hypothalamic tumours, and in later years, it has further expanded to include obesity due to other defects (such as genetic, inflammatory, head injury, cranial radiotherapy, and drug-induced defects) in hypothalamic energy-regulating pathways [3, 4] (table 1).

Early clinical and basic work in this area identified the ventromedial hypothalamus (VMH) as a critical region involved in energy homeostasis. Later, it was revealed that besides the VMH, the paraventricular nucleus (PVN), arcuate nucleus (ARC) and lateral hypothalamic area are involved in energy regulation, and damage to these areas could cause HyOb. The ARC contains two sets of neurons; one generates orexigenic responses via the agouti-related protein and neuropeptide Y, and the other generates anorexigenic responses via pro-opiomelanocortin (POMC) and cocaine- and amphetamine-related transcript. POMC is a precursor for α-melanocyte-stimulating hormone (α-MSH), which mainly affects weight regulation through the melanocortin-4 receptor (MC4R) [5]. The PVN expresses both MC4R and various Y receptors and secretes neuropeptides, including corticotrophin-releasing hormone and oxytocin, which have anorexigenic effects. Monogenic disorders of these components lead to morbid obesity, signifying their non-redundancy.

Hypothalamic damage in patients with HyOb can compromise many additional functions of the hypothalamus, which may result in hypomobility, somnolence and secondary hypopituitarism with growth hormone (GH) deficiency, hypogonadotrophic hypogonadism, secondary adrenal insufficiency, central hypothyroidism, and diabetes insipidus [6]. Monogenic HyOb is often accompanied by selective hypothalamic deficiencies, such as hypogonadotrophic hypogonadism and mild hypothalamic hypothyroidism due to leptin deficiency and hypogonadotrophic hypogonadism, GH deficiency and hypothalamic hypothyroidism due to leptin receptor deficiency [7].

Many psychotropic drugs, including several antidepressants, mood stabilisers, and antipsychotic and antiepileptic drugs, induce weight gain. The mechanism of weight gain is likely related to agonist and antagonist effects on neurotransmitter signalling in pathways that are involved in weight regulation [8]. Indeed, recent studies have confirmed the specific roles of neurotransmitters, including gamma-aminobutyric acid [9], dopamine [10], serotonin [11] and histamine [12], in hypothalamic weight control. Some of these drugs also directly increase peripheral insulin resistance and/or ß-cell insulin secretion, which can contribute to HyOb.

Fat-Brain Crosstalk: Adipocytokines

In recent years, the 'adipocytokines', which include a large number of signalling molecules that are secreted by adipose tissue, have been discovered. The secretory products of adipocytes signal energy storage and satiety to the brain and/or are involved in metabolic, inflammatory and other adipose tissue responses [13]. Leptin, which is the *ob* gene product, sends signals pertaining to body fat content to the hypothalamus. Leptin serum levels seem to directly signal information regarding energy status to regions of the central nervous system that regulate food-seeking behaviour and food intake, such as the ARC of the hypothalamus. High body fat content coincides with high leptin serum concentrations. Relative leptin resistance seems to be a critical feature of common obesity, which also leads to insulin resistance, resulting in type 2 diabetes in obese subjects [14]. New information has indicated that in humans, serum concentrations of leptin and its soluble receptor may reflect energy status and be particularly sensitive to energy deficiency states rather than reflecting satiety and be responsive to energy overload. Importantly, leptin and soluble leptin receptor have even been implicated in the pathogenesis of HyOb in children by some authors [15].

The roles of other adipocytokines, such as adiponectin, resistin, visfatin, vaspin, and chemerin, in HyOb are largely unknown. Adipocytokine serum concentrations in children and adolescents with HyOb have been reported to be low, normal or even elevated according to fat mass. These findings were obtained from data comparing concentrations in patients with so-called common obesity unrelated to a known hypothalamic pathology.

Adiponectin serum concentrations are low in obese subjects, particularly in insulin-resistant patients. Adiponectin and its receptors, AdipoR1 and AdipoR2, constitute integral components of energy homeostatic mechanisms in peripheral tissues. The presence of AdipoR1 in the hypothalamus and nucleus basalis of Meynert suggests that adiponectin may participate in the central neural signalling pathways controlling energy homeostasis [13].

Pathophysiology of Hypothalamic Obesity

When circulating leptin derived from adipocyte energy stores transduces its hypothalamic signal, an anorexigenic effect is achieved, which results in the following: (a) an increase in sympathetic tone with a resultant increase in energy expenditure; and (b) a decrease in vagal tone with resultant decreases in appetite and energy storage. Conversely, defective leptin signalling leads to an orexigenic effect, with a decrease in sympathetic tone and an increase in vagal tone and with resultant increases in appetite and energy storage [16]. Four different phenomena can disrupt leptin signalling as follows:

(a) *Leptin Deficiency.* Approximately 14 such patients have been described worldwide, who are primarily of Pakistani and Turkish descent and are largely products of consanguinity. These patients manifest hyperphagia from birth with documentable obesity as early as 6 months of age. The diagnosis is made by demonstrating extremely low or unmeasurable serum leptin levels. However, treatment with recombinant leptin is effective in restoring leptin signalling, resulting in a reduction in hyperphagia, the resolution of obesity, the induction of puberty, and the restoration of immune regulation [17].

(b) *Genetic Defects of Leptin Signal Transduction.* These disorders prevent adequate leptin signalling at either the receptor or through its second messengers and include the following: a leptin receptor mutation, POMC splicing mutation, prohormone convertase-1 deficiency, melanocortin-3 receptor mutation, MC4R mutation, and SIM1 mutation. For the most part, these disorders manifest extremely high leptin levels [14]. Currently, no treatment has been identified for these disorders.

(c) *Anatomic Defects Interfering with Leptin Signal Transduction.* Termed 'hypothalamic obesity', the death of VMH neurons prevents the integration of afferent leptin signalling; thus, the patient cannot experience a sense of energy sufficiency or a subjective state of satiety. Children with HyOb exhibit weight gain, which even occurs in response to forced caloric restriction [16]. HyOb is a therefore a manifestation of 'organic leptin resistance'.

(d) *Functional Defects in Leptin Signal Transduction.* This is postulated to be the cause of common obesity because the patient is hyperleptinaemic yet remains hungry and does not increase sympathetic tone to alter energy expenditure. These patients do not have an anatomic central nervous system defect and therefore manifest apparent 'functional leptin resistance' [18]. However, it has been recently shown that obesity due to a high-fat diet in rodents is associated with hypothalamic injury manifested by gliosis in the mediobasal hypothalamus, and similar gliosis has been found in MRI scans of the mediobasal hypothalamus of obese humans [19].

The disruption of leptin signalling in HyOb is associated with increased vagal tone, resulting in insulin hypersecretion, which is evident on oral glucose tolerance tests as shown by Bray and Gallheger [20]. Lustig et al. hypothesised that the suppression of ß-cell insulin release should promote weight loss, despite the presence of 'organic leptin resistance'. They examined the effects of the somatostatin analogue octreotide (an agonist of the somatostatin-5 receptor on ß-cells that is coupled to and inhibits voltage-gated calcium channels) in children with HyOb. A pilot, open-label trial assessing the administration of 15 µg/kg/day of octreotide subcutaneously for 6 months in 8 subjects [21] demonstrated body mass index (BMI) loss commensurate with the degree of insulin suppression along with a decrease in caloric intake and subjective improvements in spontaneous physical activity and quality of life. A double-blind, placebo-controlled trial of 20 subjects [22] resulted in insulin suppression and the stabilisation of BMI along with decreased caloric intake, increased spontaneous physical activity and an improvement in quality of life commensurate with the degree of insulin suppression. In other words, the suppression of insulin secretion promoted weight loss while improving hunger, fatigue, and malaise.

Hypothalamic Obesity in Childhood Craniopharyngioma

Childhood craniopharyngiomas (CPs) are sellar embryogenic malformations of low-grade histological malignancy and low incidence (0.5–2.0/million/year) [23]. Despite high survival rates (92%), quality of life is frequently impaired due to sequelae caused by HyOb (fig. 1). The clinical picture of CP at diagnosis is often dominated by headache and nausea, leading to further manifestations, including visual impairment (62–84%) and endocrine deficits (52–87%). A study of the history of CP patients revealed that initial symptoms, such as growth retardation and weight increase, often occur long before the diagnosis is made. Patients at risk for the development of HyOb presented with a higher BMI at the time of diagnosis in comparison to patients who maintained long-term normal weight.

For favourably localised tumours (i.e. those within the sella turcica), the first choice of treatment is an attempt at complete resection with the preservation of visual and hypothalamic functions. For unfavourably localised tumours with hypothalamic involvement, a radical surgical strategy is not recommended due to the risk of surgically induced hypothalamic deficits. After subtotal resection, the residual tumour shows progression in 71–90% of patients. The rate of progression after incomplete resection followed by radiotherapy is 21%, indicating that irradiation is efficient in the prevention of progression. Indeed, many neurosurgeons now favour stereotactic biopsy with radiation as the initial treatment of such tumours [23].

Neuropsychological Deficits: Memory, attention, impulse control, motivation, and socialisation problems have been seen as a result of the hypothalamic involvement of CP. Deficits in functional capacities depend on tumour size and extent of hypothalamic involvement.

Endocrine Deficits: Most patients (85–95%) suffer from multiple deficits of hypothalamic-pituitary function, ranging to panhypopituitarism. A full restoration of preoperatively deficient hormonal function occurs after CP resection only in exceptional cases. Irreversible diabetes insipidus follows 80–93% of all complete resections, and GH deficiency occurs in 75% of cases. The safety and effectiveness of a substitution therapy with recombinant GH has been well documented [reviewed in 23].

Hypothalamic Obesity: Obesity and eating disorders are observed in 40–50% of CP patients after surgery. Roth et al. [24] measured serum leptin levels in CP patients and found an elevated leptin concentration in relation to BMI in patients with a suprasellar tumour component. They proposed that the normal inhibition of appetite fails to occur because of a disruption in the negative feedback loop in which leptin, which is formed in adipocytes, binds to hypothalamic leptin receptors. Accelerometric measurements have shown that CP patients have a markedly lower than normal level of

Fig. 1. Central regulation of leptin signalling, autonomic innervation of adipocyte and ß-cells, and the starvation response. **a** The arcuate nucleus transduces the peripheral leptin signal, indicating a sufficiency or deficiency. In conditions of leptin sufficiency, efferents from the hypothalamus synapse in the locus coeruleus stimulate the sympathetic nervous system. In conditions of leptin deficiency, efferents from the hypothalamus stimulate the dorsal motor nucleus of the vagus. **b** Autonomic innervation and hormonal stimulation of white adipose tissue. In conditions of leptin sufficiency, norepinephrine binds to the β_3-adrenergic receptor, which stimulates hormone-sensitive lipase, promoting the lipolysis of stored triglycerides into free fatty acids. In conditions of leptin deficiency, vagal acetylcholine increases adipose tissue insulin sensitivity (documented only in rats to date), promotes the uptake of glucose and free fatty acids for lipogenesis, and promotes triglyceride uptake through the activation of lipoprotein lipase. **c** Autonomic innervation and hormonal stimulation of the β-cell. Glucose entering the cell is converted to glucose-6-phosphate by the enzyme glucokinase, generating ATP, which leads to the closing of an ATP-dependent potassium channel, resulting in cell depolarisation. A voltage-gated calcium channel opens, allowing for intracellular calcium influx, which activates neurosecretory mechanisms, leading to insulin vesicular exocytosis. In conditions of leptin sufficiency, norepinephrine binds to α_2-adrenoceptors on the β-cell membrane to stimulate inhibitory G proteins and decrease adenyl cyclase and its product cAMP, thereby reducing protein kinase A levels and insulin release. In conditions of leptin deficiency, the vagus stimulates insulin secretion through three mechanisms as follows: first, acetylcholine binds to an M_3 muscarinic receptor, opening a sodium channel, which augments ATP-dependent cell depolarisation, increasing calcium influx and insulin exocytosis. Second, acetylcholine activates a pathway that leads to an increase in protein kinase C, which also promotes insulin secretion. Third, the vagus innervates L-cells of the small intestine, which secrete glucagon-like peptide-1, activating protein kinase A and contributing to insulin exocytosis. Octreotide binds to a somatostatin receptor on the β-cell that is coupled to a voltage-gated calcium channel, limiting calcium influx and the amount of insulin released in response to glucose [24] (reprinted with kind permission by Humana, Totowa, NJ, USA). α_2-AR = α_2-adrenergic receptor; β_3-AR = β_3-adrenergic receptor; AC = adenyl cyclase; ACh = acetylcholine; DAG = diacylglycerol; DMV = dorsal motor nucleus of the vagus; FFA = free fatty acids; G_i = inhibitory G protein; GK = glucokinase; GLP-1 = glucagon-like peptide-1; GLP-1R = GLP-1 receptor; Glu-6-PO_4 = glucose-6-phosphate; Glut4 = glucose transporter-4; HSL = hormone-sensitive lipase; IML = intermediolateral cell column; IP_3 = inositol triphosphate; LC = locus coeruleus; LHA = lateral hypothalamic area; LPL = lipoprotein lipase; MARCKS = myristoylated alanine-rich protein kinase C substrate; NE = norepinephrine; PIP_2 = phosphatidylinositol; PKA = protein kinase A; PKC = protein kinase C; PLC = phospholipase C; PVN = paraventricular nucleus; $SSTR_5$ = somatostatin-5 receptor; TG = triglyceride; V_{Ca} = voltage-gated calcium channel; VMH = ventromedial hypothalamus; SUR = sulfonylurea receptor [4]. From Nature Publishing Group, with permission.

(For figure see next page.)

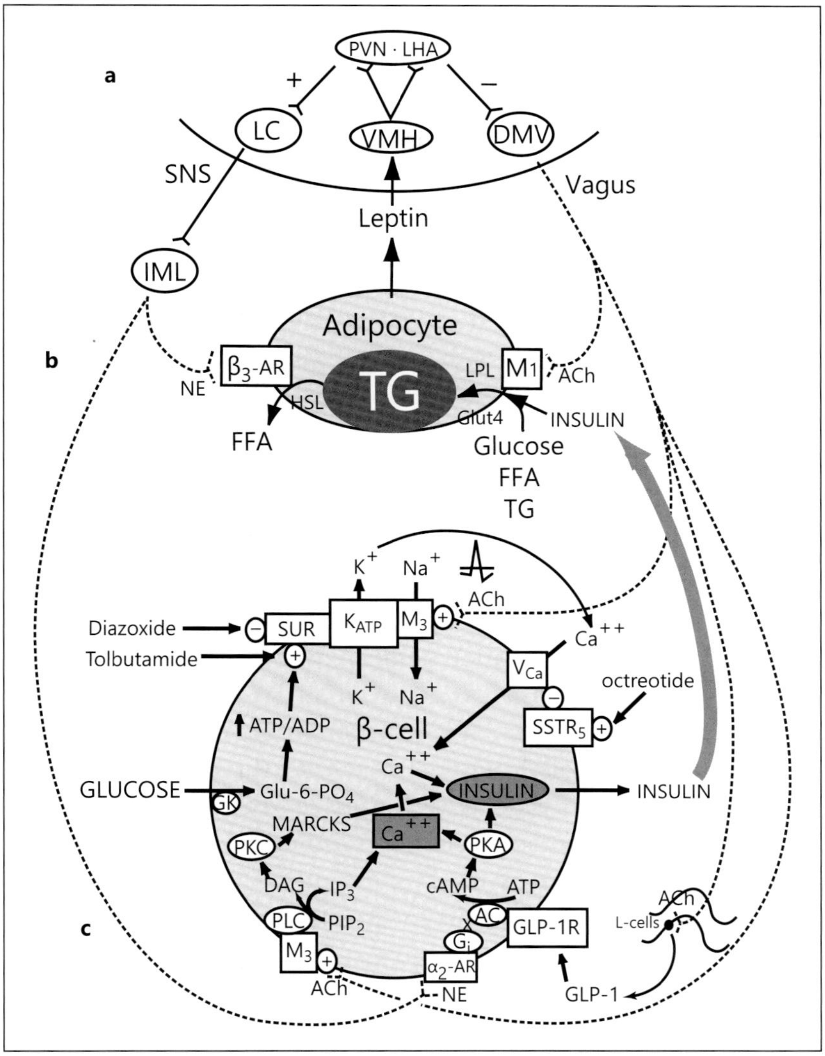

1

physical activity. Based on self-assessments using nutritional diaries, caloric intake was found to be similar in CP patients and BMI-matched controls [25]. Marked daytime sleepiness and disturbances in the circadian rhythm have been demonstrated in obese CP patients. Daytime sleepiness and obesity in these patients have both been correlated with low nocturnal melatonin levels; the proposed pathogenic mechanism involves the impaired hypothalamic regulation of circadian melatonin rhythms in patients with suprasellar CP. The first studies of melatonin substitution in patients with childhood CP, reduced melatonin levels and daytime sleepiness have shown promising results [26]. Polysomnographic studies in patients with CP and severe daytime sleepiness have revealed sleeping patterns typical of secondary narcolepsy. Notably, recent research has suggested the involvement of a hypothalamic disorder in narcolepsy. A defect in the orexin II receptor is responsible for canine narcolepsy, and orexin knockout mice show characteristic features of this disorder. Orexin is expressed exclusively in the lateral hypothalamus, and its receptors seem to be more widespread. In a study of human narcoleptics, 8 of 10 had an orexin A level that was below the detection limit of the assay [26].

Reports on the beneficial effects of treatments with central stimulating agents (modafinil and methylphenidate) have supported the hypothesis that secondary narcolepsy should be considered as a rare cause of severe daytime sleepiness in these patients [26]. Lustig et al. have postulated that the hypothalamic disinhibition of vagal output is a cause of increased ß-cell stimulation, leading to hyperinsulinism and obesity. In a double-blinded study, treatment with a somatostatin analogue (octreotide) to suppress ß-cell activity resulted in weight stabilisation [22]. Roth et al. [27] have hypothesised that decreased physical activity and severe obesity in patients with childhood CP could be related to decreased central sympathetic output. Reduced concentrations of catecholamine metabolites in the urine of patients with childhood CP correlated with the degree of obesity and the level of physical activity. α-MSH and ghrelin have been recently reported as potential pathogenic factors for HyOb in CP [28]. Analyses of ghrelin and α-MSH in a cohort of CP patients has revealed lower levels at baseline and after standard meal provocation compared to BMI-matched patients with and without other diseases responsible for obesity. It is likely that in the case of suprasellar extension, hypothalamic function is compromised and will likely remain compromised to a certain extent following treatment with surgery or irradiation. Considering the large proportion of patients with damage to the suprasellar structures, one might argue that CP and/or the effects of its treatment may result in damage to the suprachiasmatic nucleus. This may result in the altered regulation of central clock mechanisms, which predisposes patients to alterations in metabolism due to orexin pathways relevant for circadian rhythm and metabolism.

With the aid of imaging studies, recent reports have indicated that the degree of obesity of affected patients is positively correlated with the degree and extent of hypothalamic damage [29].

Despite the availability of promising therapeutic approaches, it must be emphasised that there is currently no pharmacological therapy for the treatment of obesity in CP that has been shown to be effective in controlled studies. Surgical strategies to preserve hypothalamic integrity are mandatory for the prevention of HyOb. The appropriate time point of irradiation after incomplete resection is currently under investigation.

Prader-Willi Syndrome

Prader-Willi syndrome (PWS) is a genetic neurodevelopmental disorder due to loss of paternally expressed, maternally imprinted genes within a critical chromosomal region of 15q11-q13 with a birth incidence of approximately 1:30,000 [reviewed in 30,

31]. These genes are widely expressed in the brain, including the hypothalamus. PWS arises either from a deletion of the paternal allele, maternal uniparental disomy or more rarely, from balanced translocations, imprinting control defects or microdeletions of this chromosomal region involving the paternal allele. This results in a number of neuroendocrine abnormalities, including hyperphagia and morbid obesity, hypogonadism and GH deficiency as well as characteristic facial features, developmental delay, learning difficulties and behavioural problems. By contrast, loss of the maternal *UBE3A* gene in this chromosomal region through a maternal deletion or paternal uniparental disomy results in Angelman syndrome, with clinical features that include development delay, movement disorder, characteristic behaviours, including frequent laughing, and epilepsy.

PWS has several distinct nutritional phases that occur during its natural history. First, *in utero* growth restriction with decreased foetal movements and reduced birth weight is observed (Phase 0). During Phase 1, the infant is hypotonic, initially presenting with difficulties in feeding with or without failure to thrive (sub-phase 1a), and then steady growth occurs along a growth curve, with weight increasing at a normal rate (sub-phase 1b, onset 0.4–1.3 years [25th–75th percentile]). Weight gain occurs during Phase 2, initially without a significant change in appetite or caloric intake (sub-phase 2a, onset 1.7–2.6 years), followed by an increasing interest in food (sub-phase 2b, 3.0–5.3 years). During Phase 3, there is more marked hyperphagia, which is typically accompanied by an increase in food-seeking behaviours and a lack of satiety (5–13 years). At this stage, although there is variability in the severity of the phenotype, people with PWS describe delayed meal termination, an early return of hunger after a previous meal with early meal initiation, the consumption of approximately three times the amount of food consumed by control subjects when given free access to food, the ability to eat food from the garbage and other inedible sources, the gaining of a considerable amount of weight over a short period of time if left unsupervised and the experiencing of temper tantrums related to food.

The explanation of the changes in eating behaviour and the delayed onset of hyperphagia in PWS compared to other genetic causes of hyperphagia (e.g. leptin deficiency, SIM1 deletions or MC4R mutations) remains unclear but might be more related to normal, abnormal or delayed brain development than changes in peripheral signals, such as appetitive gut hormones.

The marked propensity for excessive eating that continues throughout life causes significant morbidity and mortality in PWS. Type 2 diabetes mellitus has been reported in approximately 25% of adults with PWS (mean age of onset of approximately 20 years) and hypertension has been described in up to 38% of adults, although it is uncommon in children [30]. Interestingly, MRI analysis has found a selective relative reduction in visceral adiposity in non-diabetic PWS adults. This may explain the relative preservation of insulin sensitivity, protective elevation in adiponectin levels, and normal triglyceride levels in PWS patients given their overall obesity. The use of lipid-lowering therapy may therefore be required less frequently than might be expected. Death in PWS adults is most often obesity-related and due to cardiorespiratory failure, cor pulmonale exacerbated by obstructive and central apnoea, septicaemia due to skin infections, and pneumonia.

The normal feedback mechanisms that result in the metabolic and neuropsychological (loss of hunger) changes associated with food intake are impaired in PWS. Studies of eating behaviour, appetitive gut hormones, structural and functional brain imaging and post-mortem studies have revealed a number of potential neuroendocrine phenotypes that may contribute to hyperphagia and obesity in PWS. Potentially causative phenotypes are a low plasma level of the anorexigenic hormone pancreatic polypeptide, high plasma level of the orexigenic stomach-derived hormone ghrelin, and low oxytocin cell number in the hypothalamic PVN. However, their relative roles, relationships with the evolution of childhood eating behaviours, links to specific PWS genes and hence, the suitability of their targeting for potential treatments remains unclear.

Previous studies have consistently shown that fasting plasma ghrelin levels are raised in older children (after the usual age of development of hyperphagia) and adults with PWS relative to their obesity levels. Up to 3- to 4-fold increases in ghrelin have been reported in PWS patients compared with controls after adjusting for BMI or body composition, and some studies using lean controls have shown even higher elevations [30, 32]. Levels of ghrelin fall after food intake in children and adults with PWS but remain elevated compared to obese controls. Elevations in the active acylated form of ghrelin have also been reported in PWS [32]. Increased numbers of ghrelin-expressing cells have been reported in the gastric body and fundus of these patients. There is contradictory evidence as to whether hyperghrelinaemia does or does not precede or even coincide with the development of hyperphagia in PWS children. Interestingly, plasma pancreatic polypeptide levels do appear to be reduced even before the onset of hyperphagia in PWS. Other possible causes of the elevated ghrelin levels observed in PWS include abnormal parasympathetic vagal innervation of the stomach and sympathetic tone [30].

Obesity management in PWS patients involves the following: (i) early diagnosis, allowing for the early institution of a low-calorie, well-balanced diet; (ii) appropriate psychological and behavioural counselling of the patient and family; (iii) early, repeated discussions of the inevitability of hyperphagia (even in infancy); (iv) the vigorous supervision and control of the food environment; (v) the restriction of access to food and money with appreciation of legal and ethical obligations; (vi) regular exercise (physical activity is reduced in PWS patients due to obesity, hypersomnolence and persistent poor muscle tone, while resting metabolic rate relative to body size is reduced due to abnormal body composition); and (vii) GH therapy, which helps to reduce fat mass and increase muscle mass, although there is no evidence that it results in the alteration of hyperphagia [31].

There is no evidence of benefits to patients acquired from the pharmacological treatment of hyperphagia, including the use of anorexigenic agents, such as sibutramine, dexfenfluramine or topiramate, although there are few published placebo-controlled studies [31]. While a recent study has shown some efficacy for the endocannabinoid CB1 receptor antagonist rimonabant, it is associated with unacceptable psychiatric side effects [33]. The acute or long-term suppression of ghrelin secretion using somatostatin and its analogues has no benefit on overeating, but an investigation of ghrelin antagonists or acylating enzyme that activates ghrelin inhibitors should be performed before concluding that targeting the ghrelin pathway is of no benefit for the treatment of PWS [31]. A recent study of the glucagon-like peptide 1 (GLP-1) agonist exenatide in PWS patients has shown that it acutely increases satiety and exerts glucose-lowering and insulinotropic effects [34]. The safety and tolerability of GLP-1 agonists in patients with PWS is however unknown. One theoretical concern is its effects on gastric motility. Gastric emptying is delayed in people with PWS. GLP-1 agonists may further delay gastric emptying (contributing to their beneficial effects on satiety and glycaemic control), and indeed, diabetic gastroparaesis is a contraindication for their use. Therefore, appropriate investigations of their safety and efficacy need to be performed in this patient group before they are widely used as new treatments for diabetes and/or weight loss in PWS.

Bariatric surgery, e.g. gastric banding or bypass, is not considered to reduce overeating or produce long-term weight reduction and is associated with high morbidity and mortality [35]. Unlike other obese patients, those with PWS typically have several defects that may alter the rate and severity of and even hide the clinical presentation of bariatric surgery complications, including reduced satiety, an increased pain threshold, autonomic dysfunction, delayed gastric emptying and a decreased ability to vomit, skin picking and sleep-disordered breathing. For example, these factors are likely to have contributed to the higher-than-expected rates of gastric distension, perforation and obstruction that were reported as a result of a series of intragastric balloon placements in patients with PWS despite close outpatient nutritional monitoring to restrict food access. Thus, the current expert opinion is that there is little justification for subjecting PWS patients to the potential risks of surgical interventions. The use of supervised reduced-energy diets with vitamin/mineral supplementation, tight restrictions on food access in a controlled environment dedicated to the management of patients with PWS, and a daily exercise regimen are preferred.

Pharmacological Treatment of Hypothalamic Obesity

HyOb is usually progressive and unresponsive to conventional lifestyle modifications (diet and exercise) (fig. 2). There is no standard pharmacological intervention that has consistently been shown to have a positive effect in these complicated patients. Several agents have been used to treat HyOb for limited periods, yet it is difficult to compare the effects of such interventions that have been used for different periods and at different time points of obesity development following the hypothalamic insult. The

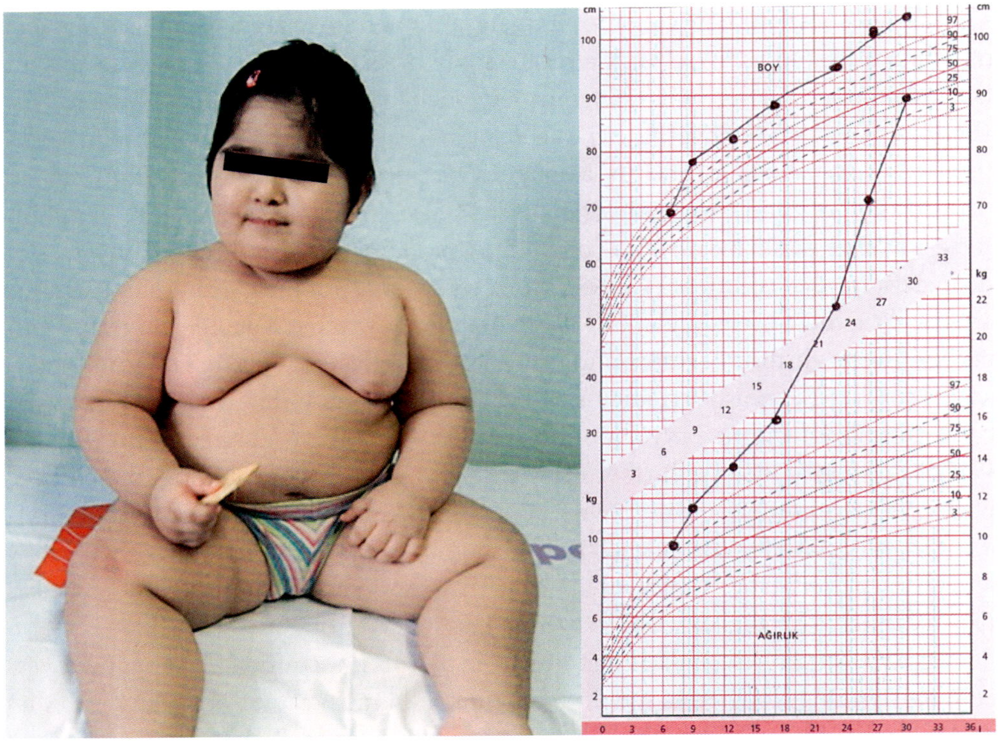

Fig. 2. A 2.5-year-old girl with hypothalamic obesity due to a hypothalamic tumour. A progressive increase in weight is indicated on her growth chart.

vast majority of the studies described herein were performed on a very small number of patients; thus, generalised conclusions that can be applied to other patients with HyOb may be limited.

Based on the observation that patients with HyOb demonstrate impairments in sympatho-adrenal activation and epinephrine production manifesting as a reduced hormonal response to hypoglycaemia, treating this disorder with amphetamine derivatives has been suggested. The use of dextroamphetamine beginning at 10 months post-surgical intervention for CP up until 24 months has been shown to diminish continuous weight gain and stabilise BMI [36]. Importantly, spontaneous physical activity has been demonstrated to significantly increase. Shorter periods of dextroamphetamine treatment have been shown to cause a subjective improvement in daytime wakefulness. Similar results have been reported with an ephedrine/caffeine mixture [reviewed in 5].

Weight loss in HyOb patients on sibutramine treatment in a controlled cross-over trial has been shown to be less pronounced in comparison with other groups of obese participants (such as those with trisomy 21 and PWS), manifesting as 'partial resistance' to the intervention [37]. While its effect on BMI SD scores was promising, this drug has been taken off the market; thus, its future use in clinical trials is not expected.

Patients with HyOb have a 'parasympathetic predominance' of the autonomic nervous system induced by vagal activation and manifesting as tiredness, slow pulse and reduced body temperature. Parasympathetic stimulation causes insulin secretion by way of the direct activation of β-cells as well as the promotion of adipogenesis. Because insulin is an anabolic hormone, it has been suggested to be an important driver of weight gain in HyOb patients. Octreotide is a somatostatin analogue that causes a reduction in insulin secretion. Lustig et al. have used octreotide in a double-blind, randomised controlled study in children with HyOb, demonstrating significant reductions in weight gain and BMI [22]. As a proof of concept, the authors have shown that insulin levels during an oral glucose tolerance test decrease significantly without leading to major changes in glucose tolerance. This study was followed by a larger multinational one performed to assess the use of octreotide long-acting repeatable in 60 patients with cranial surgical interventions that led to HyOb [38]. The intervention was 6 months in duration and showed no efficacy at all according to the primary end-point of change in BMI. However, the placebo-treated group did not gain weight during this trial. It is important to note that the two studies described differ in the crucial issue of timing, i.e. when the intervention was introduced. Patients with HyOb typically gain weight rapidly during the first months following the hypothalamic insult, and this phase is followed by a slower weight gain pattern. While Lustig et al. introduced their intervention early, it seems that the octreotide long-acting repeatable study was performed during a later phase of HyOb development. Thus, it is difficult to compare these studies and draw definitive conclusions regarding the use of octreotide derivatives in the context of HyOb. The open-label segment of the Lustig et al. study was terminated earlier than planned due to an increased risk of gallstone formation.

Based on the hormonal milieu demonstrated in patients with HyOb, several researchers have attempted to address hormonal defects exogenously. The typical 'parasympathetic dominance' observed in patients with HyOb also manifests as reduced T_3 levels. This information led researchers to provide T_3 supplementation to patients with HyOb. Although only 3 patients were evaluated, the authors reported significant weight loss and improved alertness in these participants [39]. Tiosano et al. demonstrated increased 11β-hydroxysteroid dehydrogenase-1 activity in patients with HyOb [40]. They proposed that a deficiency in hypothalamic messengers after surgical injury induces a paracrine/autocrine effect of enhanced glucocorticoid activity due to up-regulated 11β-HSD1 activity. This finding obviously suggests that the inhibition of this enzyme may have therapeutic advantages in this context; however, a selective inhibitor is at present only in development. Because patients with HyOb may present with GH deficiency (despite seemingly normal 'growth without GH'), treatment with GHs has also been attempted in this unique group. Unlike patients with GH deficiency due to other causes, patients with HyOb do not exhibit slowed weight and BMI gains with GH therapy [41]. Recently, the GLP-1 analogue treatment of nine adults with HyOb for up to 51 months was shown to cause substantial weight loss (–13.1 ± 5.1 kg, range: –9 to –22). Insulin resistance and HbA1c values improved under this treatment. Five patients reported increased satiation in response to the treatment. Two of the eight patients complained of nausea and vomiting, and one abandoned the therapy because of sustained gastrointestinal discomfort after 6 months. One patient suffered from intolerable nausea and vomiting and discontinued treatment within 2 weeks. Thus, it seems that GLP-1 analogues offer a new approach for the medical treatment of moderate to severe HyOb and associated metabolic alterations [42].

Considering the above described studies, there is presently no 'magic bullet' for addressing HyOb in children. The conclusion that one can draw from the studies performed thus far is that timing is a major issue in designing effective future interventions for this complex condition. This means that any such interventions should be administered as close as possible to the surgical insult and prior to the massive early weight gain. Because multiple hormonal deficiencies and aberrations have been described in the context of HyOb, it would make sense to combine several treatment modalities to address the multiple processes driving weight gain in these patients.

Bariatric Surgery in the Management of Hypothalamic Obesity in Children and Adolescents

Bariatric surgery is a last resort and is rarely performed on obese adolescent patients. A systematic literature search (1955–2013) identified 637 adolescent patients from 23 studies who showed significant decreases in BMI at 1 year (average weighted mean BMI difference: –13.5) [43]. The risks of complications are not well defined in the literature.

HyOb is a relatively rare form of obesity; thus, controlled randomised trials in this specific group of patients are lacking. However, first experiences with bariatric surgery (gastric banding) to treat severe obesity after childhood CP in children are encouraging [44].

The following guidelines [45] have been suggested for childhood bariatric surgery: if the patient

(1) has a BMI of >40 (or the 99.5th percentile for the respective age) and at least one co-morbidity,

(2) has failed at least 6–12 months of organised weight loss attempts at a specialised centre,

(3) shows skeletal and developmental maturity,

(4) is able to commit to comprehensive medical and psychological evaluations before and after surgery,

(5) is willing to participate in a post-operative multidisciplinary treatment program, and

(6) has access to a surgery unit with specialised paediatric support.

The aforementioned criteria also apply to adolescents or adults with HyOb but must be considered carefully in younger patients, who less-frequently fulfil all of the requirements. Successful bariatric surgery can only be accomplished by active participation and understanding and the consent of both the patient and any relevant caregivers.

Bariatric procedures are performed either to reduce appetite, restrict the amount of food intake or deploy malabsorption; however, for the combined technique, the former and latter methods are merged. Gastric banding, sleeve gastrectomy, and laparoscopic greater curvature plication are among the restrictive procedures performed. Gastric bypass and duodenal switch/biliopancreatic diversion are among the malabsorptive procedures performed.

Gastric bypass involves creating a small gastric pouch of less than 30 ml and Roux-en-Y anastomosis. One advantage of bypass is that it may decrease or prevent a weight loss-associated rise in plasma ghrelin levels. Sugerman et al. [46] reported a series of 32 children with a mean age of 16 ± 1 years (range: 12.4–17.9 years) who underwent various operations, including gastric bypass. The overall excess weight loss was 33% for a mean follow-up time of 11 years and an 18% 'failure' rate, which was defined as the total weight regain. There are case reports describing the successful management of adolescents with this technique [47]. In a series involving duodenal switch/biliopancreatic diversion performed on 13 adolescents ranging in age from 15 to 17 years who were followed up for 2–16 years, no important side effects or deficiencies were reported, except for marginally low levels of vitamins that required supplements [48]. The largest series performed on adolescents (n = 68) with the longest follow-up time (mean of 11 [range: 2–23] years) was reported in 2007 by Papadia et al. [49]. They reported a 78% excess weight loss at the cost of protein deficiency (16%), reoperations (13%), and increased long-term mortality (5%). A recent review of the effects of bariatric surgery on obesity after CP in adults identified a total of 21 cases, including 6 with adjustable gastric banding, 8 with sleeve gastrectomy, 6 with Roux-en-Y gastric bypass, and 1 with biliopancreatic diversion. The mean weight difference was –20.9 kg after 6 months and –15.1 kg after 12 months [50]. Such data in adolescents are still lacking.

Bariatric surgery leads to serious complications, including death, deep venous thrombosis and pulmonary embolism, gastrojejunal anastomotic leak, gastrojejunal anastomotic stricture, bleeding, gastric remnant dilatation, jejunojejunostomy obstruction, internal hernia, marginal (jejunal) ulcer, adhesive small-bowel obstruction, port-site small bowel obstruction, nausea, vomiting, and dehydration.

Nutritional deficiencies after malabsorptive procedures include iron and vitamin B12 deficiency, which are related to reduced acid and intrinsic factor production, vitamin D/calcium deficiencies, thiamine deficiency, folate deficiency, and hyperinsulinaemic hypoglycaemia. Thus, patients should be supplemented with these vitamins after bariatric surgery.

Among the novel bariatric interventions, vagal blockade may be a promising method in the treatment of HyOb because increased vagal tone is one of the mechanisms underlying increased food intake and energy storage. The idea of blocking the vagus has stemmed from studies utilising vagotomy alone or in combination with other bariatric procedures to treat obesity [51]. It has been shown in obese rodents that the action of hypothalamic leptin increases peripheral insulin sensitivity primarily via effects on the liver and that the mechanism underlying this effect is dependent upon the hepatic branch of the vagus nerve. Furthermore, the food deprivation-induced elevations in plasma ghrelin levels are completely prevented by subdiaphragmatic vagotomy [52].

References

1 Babinski J: Tumeur du corps pituitaire sans acromégalie et avec arrêt de développement des organes génitaux. Rev Neurol 1900;8:531–533.

2 Frohlich A: Ein fall von tumor der hypophysis cerebri ohne akromegalie. Wiener Klin Rdsch 1901;15:883–886.

3 Hochberg I, Hochberg Z: Expanding the definition of hypothalamic obesity. Obes Rev 2010;11:709–721.

4 Bereket A, Kiess W, Lustig RH, et al: Hypothalamic obesity in children. Obes Rev 2012;13:780–798.

5 Coll AP, Farooqi IS, Challis BG, Yeo GS, O'Rahilly S: Proopiomelanocortin and energy balance: insights from human and murine genetics. J Clin Endocrinol Metab 2004;89:2557–2562.

6 Snow A, Gozal E, Malhotra A, et al: Severe hypersomnolence after pituitary/hypothalamic surgery in adolescents: clinical characteristics and potential mechanisms. Pediatrics 2002;110:e74.

7 Clement K, Vaisse C, Lahlou N, et al: A mutation in the human leptin receptor gene causes obesity and pituitary dysfunction. Nature 1998;392:398–401.

8 Zimmermann U, Kraus T, Himmerich H, Schuld A, Pollmacher T: Epidemiology, implications and mechanisms underlying drug-induced weight gain in psychiatric patients. J Psychiatr Res 2003;37:193–220.

9 Tong Q, Ye CP, Jones JE, Elmquist JK, Lowell BB: Synaptic release of GABA by AgRP neurons is required for normal regulation of energy balance. Nat Neurosci 2008;11:998–1000.

10 Abizaid A, Liu ZW, Andrews ZB, et al: Ghrelin modulates the activity and synaptic input organization of midbrain dopamine neurons while promoting appetite. J Clin Invest 2006;116:3229–3239.

11 Heisler LK, Jobst EE, Sutton GM, et al: Serotonin reciprocally regulates melanocortin neurons to modulate food intake. Neuron 2006;51:239–249.

12 Kim SF, Huang AS, Snowman AM, Teuscher C, Snyder SH: From the cover: antipsychotic drug-induced weight gain mediated by histamine H1 receptor-linked activation of hypothalamic AMP-kinase. Proc Natl Acad Sci USA 2007;104:3456–3459.

13 Körner A, Kratzsch J, Kiess W: Adipocytokines: leptin–the classical, resistin–the controversical, adiponectin–the promising, and more to come. Best Pract Res Clin Endocrinol Metab 2005;19:525–546.

14 Farooqi IS, O'Rahilly S: Genetics of obesity in humans. Endocr Rev 2006;27:710–718.

15 Guran T, Turan S, Bereket A, et al: The role of leptin, soluble leptin receptor, resistin, and insulin secretory dynamics in the pathogenesis of hypothalamic obesity in children. Eur J Pediatr 2009;168:1043–1048.

16 Lustig RH, Sen S, Soberman JE, Velasquez-Mieyer PA: Obesity, leptin resistance, and the effects of insulin suppression. Int J Obes 2004;28:1344–1348.

17 Farooqi IS, Jebb SA, Langmack G, et al: Effects of recombinant leptin therapy in a child with congenital leptin deficiency. New Engl J Med 1999;341:913–915.

18 Heymsfield SB, Greenberg AS, Fujioka K, et al: Recombinant leptin for weight loss in obese and lean adults: a randomized, controlled, dose-escalation trial. JAMA 1999;282:1568–1575.

19 Thaler JP, Yi CX, Schur EA, et al: Obesity is associated with hypothalamic injury in rodents and humans. J Clin Invest 2012;122:153–162.

20 Bray GA, Gallagher TF: Manifestations of hypothalamic obesity in man: a comprehensive investigation of eight patients and a review of the literature. Medicine 1975;54:301–333.

21 Lustig RH, Rose SR, Burghen GA, et al: Hypothalamic obesity in children caused by cranial insult: altered glucose and insulin dynamics, and reversal by a somatostatin agonist. J Pediatr 1999;135:162–168.

22 Lustig RH, Hinds PS, Ringwald-Smith K, et al: Octreotide therapy of pediatric hypothalamic obesity: a double-blind, placebo-controlled trial. J Clin Endocrinol Metab 2003;88:2586–2592.

23 Müller HL: Childhood craniopharyngioma – current concepts in diagnosis, therapy and follow-up. Nat Rev Endocrinol 2010;6:609–618.
24 Roth C, Wilken B, Hanefeld F, Schröter W, Leonhardt U: Hyperphagia in children with craniopharyngioma is associated with hyperleptinemia and a failure in the down regulation of appetite. Eur J Endocrinol 1998;138:89–91.
25 Harz KJ, Müller HL, Waldeck E, Pudel V, Roth C: Obesity in patients with craniopharyngioma: assessment of physical activity and food intake. J Clin Endocrinol Metab 2003;88:5227–5231.
26 Müller HL: Increased daytime sleepiness in patients with childhood craniopharyngioma and hypothalamic tumor involvement: review of the literature and perspectives. Int J Endocrinol 2010;2010: 519607.
27 Roth C, Hunneman D, Gebhardt U, Stoffel-Wagner B, Reinehr T, Müller HL: Reduced sympathetic metabolites in urine of obese patients with craniopharyngioma. Pediatr Res 2006;61:496–501.
28 Roth C, Gebhardt U, Müller HL: Appetite-regulating hormone changes in patients with craniopharyngioma. Obesity (Silver Spring) 2011;19:36–41.
29 De Vile CJ, Grant DB, Hayward RD, Kendall BE, Neville BGR, Stanhope R: Obesity in childhood craniopharyngioma: relation to post-operative hypothalamic damage shown by magnetic resonance imaging. J Clin Endocrinol Metab 1996;81:2734–2737.
30 Goldstone AP: Prader-Willi syndrome: advances in its genetics, pathophysiology and treatment. Trends Endocrinol Metab 2004;15:12–20.
31 Goldstone AP, Holland AJ, Hauffa BP, Hokken-Koelega AC, Tauber M: Recommendations for the diagnosis and management of Prader-Willi syndrome. J Clin Endocrinol Metab 2008;93:4183–4197.
32 Goldstone AP, Patterson M, Kalingag N, et al: Fasting and post-prandial hyperghrelinemia in Prader-Willi syndrome is partially explained by hypoinsulinemia, and is not due to peptide YY 3–36 deficiency or seen in hypothalamic obesity due to craniopharyngioma. J Clin Endocrinol Metab 2005; 90:2681–2690.
33 Motaghedi R, Lipman EG, Hogg JE, Christos PJ, Vogiatzi MG, Angulo MA: Psychiatric adverse effects of rimonobant in adults with Prader Willi syndrome. Eur J Med Genet 2011;54:14–18.
34 Sze L, Purtell L, Jenkins A, et al: Effects of a single dose of exenatide on appetite, gut hormones, and glucose homeostasis in adults with Prader-Willi syndrome. J Clin Endocrinol Metab 2011;96:E1314–E1319.
35 Scheimann AO, Butler MG, Gourash L, Cuffari C, Klish W: Critical analysis of bariatric procedures in Prader-Willi syndrome. J Pediatr Gastroenterol Nutr 2008;46:80–83.
36 Mason PW, Krawiecki N, Meacham LR: The use of dextroamphetamine to treat obesity and hyperphagia in children treated for craniopharyngioma. Arch Pediatr Adolesc Med 2002;156:887–892.
37 Danielsson P, Janson A, Norgren S, Marcus C: Impact of sibutramine therapy in children with hypothalamic obesity or obesity with aggravating syndromes. J Clin Endocrinol Metab 2007;92:4101–4106.
38 Lustig RH, Greenway F, Velasquez-Mieyer P, et al: A multicenter, randomized, double-blind, placebo-controlled, dose-finding trial of a long-acting formulation of octreotide in promoting weight loss in obese adults with insulin hypersecretion. Int J Obesity 2006;30:331–341.
39 Fernandes JK, Klein MJ, Ater JL, Kuttesch JF, Vassilopoulou-Sellin R: Triiodothyronine supplementation for hypothalamic obesity. Metabolism 2002;51: 1381–1383.
40 Tiosano D, Eisentein I, Militianu D, Chrousos GP, Hochberg Z: 11 beta-hydroxysteroid dehydrogenase activity in hypothalamic obesity. J Clin Endocrinol Metab 2003;88:379–384.
41 Geffner M, Lundberg M, Koltowska-Häggström M, et al: Changes in height, weight, and body mass index in children with craniopharyngioma after three years of growth hormone therapy: analysis of KIGS (Pfizer International Growth Database). J Clin Endocrinol Metab 2004 ;89:5435–5440.
42 Zoicas F, Droste M, Mayr B, Buchfelder M, Schöfl C: GLP-1 analogues as a new treatment option for hypothalamic obesity in adults: report of nine cases. Eur J Endocrinol 2013;168:699–706.
43 Black JA, White B, Viner RM, Simmons RK: Bariatric surgery for obese children and adolescents: a systematic review and meta-analysis. Obes Rev 2013;14: 634–644.
44 Müller HL, Gebhardt U, Maroske J, Hanisch E: Long-term follow-up of morbidly obese patients with childhood craniopharyngioma after laparoscopic adjustable gastric banding (LAGB). Klin Padiatr 2011;223:372–373.
45 Fried M, Hainer V, Basdevant A, et al: Bariatric Scientific Collaborative Group Expert Panel Interdisciplinary European Guidelines for surgery for severe (morbid) obesity. Obes Surg 2007;17:260–270.
46 Sugerman HJ, Sugerman EL, DeMaria EJ, et al: Bariatric surgery for severely obese adolescents. J Gastrointest Surg 2003;7:102–107.
47 Daskalakis M, Till H, Kiess W, Weiner RA: Roux-en-Y gastric bypass in an adolescent patient with Bardet-Biedl syndrome, a monogenic obesity disorder. Obes Surg 2010;20:121–125.
48 Marceau P, Marceau S, Biron S, et al: Long-term experience with duodenal switch in adolescents. Obes Surg 2010;20:1609–1616.

49 Papadia FS, Adami GF, Marinari GM, Camerini G, Scopinaro N: Bariatric surgery in adolescents: a long-term follow-up study. Surg Obes Relat Dis 2007;3:465–468.
50 Bretault M, Boillot A, Muzard L, et al: Clinical review: bariatric surgery following treatment for craniopharyngioma: a systematic review and individual-level data meta-analysis. J Clin Endocrinol Metab 2013;98:2239–2246.
51 Kral JG, Görtz L, Hermansson G, Wallin GS: Gastroplasty for obesity: long-term weight loss improved by vagotomy. World J Surg 1998;17:75–78.
52 German J, Kim F, Schwartz GJ, et al: Hypothalamic leptin signaling regulates hepatic insulin sensitivity via a neurocircuit involving the vagus nerve. Endocrinology 2009;150:4502–4511.

Abdullah Bereket, MD
Department of Paediatrics, Marmara University
Dr. Faruk Ayanoglu caddesi, No: 50/11
TR–34726 Fenerbahce-Istanbul (Turkey)
E-Mail abdullahbereket@gmail.com

Kiess W, Wabitsch M, Maffeis C, Sharma AM (eds): Metabolic Syndrome and Obesity in Childhood and Adolescence.
Pediatr Adolesc Med. Basel, Karger, 2015, vol 19, pp 31–39 (DOI: 10.1159/000368103)

Genetics of Obesity in Childhood and Adolescence

Yvonne Böttcher • Peter Kovacs

IFB AdiposityDiseases, Medical Faculty, University of Leipzig, Leipzig, Germany

Abstract

Obesity is controlled by both genetic and nongenetic factors. Considering BMI as a simple measure of obesity, heritability estimates reach 0.7 for both adults and children. Explaining the heritability of common polygenic obesity remains one of the major challenges in obesity research. Whereas candidate gene and genome-wide linkage studies dominated the search for obesity susceptibility genes over the last two decades, recent advances in genotyping technologies, enabling the high-throughput testing of millions of variants in thousands of individuals, have shown genome-wide association studies (GWASs) to be an efficient tool to identify novel loci associated with obesity. GWASs have revealed that more than 30 polymorphisms are significantly associated with obesity, including those mapping within genes such as *FTO*, *TMEM18*, and *MC4R*. Although many of these genes seem to influence childhood obesity as well, recent GWASs uncovered a strong association of novel loci (*OLFM4* and *HOXB5*) with common early-onset obesity. Future studies need to address the biological role of these novel genes in obesity's complex pathophysiology, as well as its missing heritability, since only a small proportion can be explained so far.

Introduction

Obesity is one of the major predictors of common civilization diseases such as type 2 diabetes (T2D), hypertension, cardiovascular diseases, and associated forms of cancer and thus represents a major public health burden [1]. In addition, obesity is strongly linked to psychological disorders, at least in part due to social stigmatism, which leads to further excess weight gain. Considering BMI as a simple measure of obesity, the prevalence of obesity increased rapidly during the last decade. It has been estimated that 1.12 billion adults will become obese (BMI >30) and that more than 2 billion will be overweight (BMI >25) by 2030 [2]. The epidemic proportion of obesity in adults mirrors the situation in children, among whom the incidence has increased dramatically and is expected to reach ~30% in the United States by 2030 [3]. Whereas a small proportion of obesity can clearly be attributed to monogenic forms caused by rare genetic defects, it is well appreciated that common 'epidemic' obesity is a complex polygenic disease with both genetic and environmental determinants. In particular, the adoption of a modern lifestyle, manifested by easy access to high-calorie food and accompanied by reduced energy expenditure, represents a major unfavorable environmental component that is contributing to the ongoing epidemic expansion of obesity worldwide [4, reviewed in 5].

Nevertheless, there is no doubt that obesity has genetic components. Major evidence comes from family, twin, and adoption studies, which have provided heritability estimates for BMI as high as 70% in both adults and children [6, 7]. Maternal or paternal obesity is one of the crucial predictors of an increased risk of childhood obesity, with the highest risk occurring when both parents manifest obesity [8]. Nevertheless, as for any other complex polygenic trait, obesity is clearly affected by the environment, which, in a complex interplay with genetics, may result in the disease phenotype.

The search for obesity susceptibility genes has focused on candidate gene and genome-wide strategies. Genome-wide linkage studies represented major approaches for identifying obesity genes over the last two decades. However, advances in genotyping technologies allowed the replacement of these strategies by genome-wide association studies (GWASs). Moreover, admixture mapping based on recent differences in genetic ancestries have revealed a significant relationship between ethnicity and obesity for several genetic regions [9].

This review aims to elaborate the current knowledge of the genetics of obesity.

Polygenic Obesity

Despite the knowledge gained from lessons in monogenic obesity, explaining the heritability of polygenic obesity remains a major challenge in obesity research. This challenge is attributable to the polygenic nature of common obesity as well as to the strong influence of environmental factors. Two major approaches have been used to investigate the components underlying the genetics of obesity: (i) analyses of candidate genes based on their known biological function related to regulation of metabolism and (ii) hypothesis-free genome-wide strategies, both potentially uncovering genes with yet-unknown roles in the pathophysiology of human obesity.

Candidate Gene Approach

The selection of plausible candidate genes for genetic analyses requires a priori knowledge about the pathophysiology of a disease and about the gene's/protein's function. Comprehensive studies on genes regulating energy balance and glucose/insulin metabolism resulted in numerous sequence variants that were significantly associated with obesity and related traits. Despite recent advances in high-throughput genotyping technologies, allowing the performance of large-scale genome-wide screening studies, the candidate gene approach still deserves researchers' attention. In particular, it provides an efficient tool to verify and/or to finely map the most promising regions from genome-wide efforts and to elucidate the role of rare variants potentially contributing to polygenic obesity. For instance, rare variants in two genes controlling the endocannabinoid system, the fatty acid amide hydrolase gene (*FAAH*) and the monoglyceride lipase gene *(MGLL),* were shown to be associated with extreme obesity and metabolite levels [10].

Fatty Acid Synthase Gene

Human fatty acid synthase (FASN) is the major determinant of the de novo synthesis of long-chain fatty acids from acetyl-CoA, malonyl-CoA, and NADPH [11]. Inhibition of the FASN causes a fast decrease in fat stores in mice, suggesting a role for the FASN in energy homeostasis, which makes its gene an attractive candidate for systematic genetic analyses [12]. In addition, *FASN* represents a strong positional candidate gene since it maps within a linkage region on chromosome 17q25, which was identified in a genome-wide family-based scan for obesity susceptibility genes in Pima Indians from Arizona. In subsequent fine-mapping studies, the contribution of *FASN* to human body weight and the percentage of body fat was investigated not only in Pima Indians but also in other ethnic populations [13]. A polymorphism predicting the amino acid substitution Val1348Ile has been shown to be associated with the percentage of body fat and the 24-hour substrate oxidation rate in Pima Indians [13]. Moreover, the likely protective effects of this variant against obesity have been supported by data from children and adolescents from Germany [14]. Interestingly, the polymorphism seems to have stronger effects in boys, thus suggesting sexual dimorphism in FASN action. Additionally, studies on mRNA expression that showed correlations of increased *FASN* mRNA levels in adipose tissue with visceral fat accumulation and impaired insulin sensitivity clearly suggest a role for the FASN in the pathophysiology of obesity [15]. Consistent with this finding, obesity-related FASN genetic variants have been shown to be associated with mRNA expression in visceral and subcutaneous adipose tissue [16].

Genome-Wide Strategies

Linkage Analyses

Family-based genome-wide linkage scans offer a unique tool to assess the co-segregation of highly polymorphic genetic markers with a phenotypic trait/disease. Whereas this strategy turned out to be very efficient for monogenic forms of obesity, less success has been achieved in polygenic obesity. Moreover, the associations of genetic variants with obesity that were identified in linkage studies were not replicated in subsequent efforts, thus suggesting a small increase in the risk of obesity for these common variants.

The ectonucleotide pyrophosphatase/phosphodiesterase 1 gene *(ENPP1)*, which maps to chromosome 6q, is one of the few representatives identified via genome-wide linkage analysis as linked to childhood obesity and associated traits [17]. The encoded protein ENPP1 binds to the α-subunit of the insulin receptor and inhibits its insulin-mediated conformational changes, autophosphorylation, and tyrosine kinase activity [18]. A nonsynonymous K121Q polymorphism in exon 4 of *ENPP1* has been reported to be strongly associated with insulin resistance in healthy, nonobese individuals [19]. Subsequent studies in distinct populations confirmed the associations of the K121Q variant with insulin resistance and T2D [20, 21]. Consistent with this finding, positional cloning within the chromosomal region revealed significant association of a haplotype consisting of three *ENPP1* variants (K121Q, IVS20delT-11, and A/G+1044TGA) with childhood and adult obesity and T2D [22]. In addition, obesity risk alleles were correlated with impaired glucose tolerance as well as increased serum levels of soluble ENPP1 in children [22]. Whereas the association with childhood obesity was replicated in a case-control study, no relationship between the risk alleles and BMI was observed in a population-based study with healthy Caucasian children [23]. In obese children, the risk haplotype (Q-delT-G) was accompanied by impaired glucose metabolism, whereas the (K-delT-G) and (K-insT-A) haplotypes were associated with improved insulin sensitivity and glucose metabolism [23]. Despite failure to replicate these associations in numerous individual studies, a well-powered meta-analysis including 24,324 subjects suggested that the *ENPP1* Q121 variant might increase the risk of obesity [24].

Genome-Wide Association Studies

Recent advances in technologies in molecular biology, including high-throughput genotyping techniques, have allowed researchers to employ GWASs in identifying novel loci associated with human obesity. As anticipated, GWASs have turned out to be a very powerful tool for the identification of genetic variants with a moderate effect size. However, despite very promising progress in determining the genetics of complex diseases such as obesity, even with numerous susceptibility genes revealed so far, most of the heritability of obesity is yet to be determined.

Fat Mass- and Obesity-Associated Gene

Associations of fat mass- and obesity associated gene *(FTO)* polymorphisms with common obesity were first reported in 2007 [25]. Researchers at the Wellcome Trust Case Control Consortium (WTCCC) conducted a GWAS aimed at identifying genetic determinants of T2D. Using 500K Affymetrix chips, they observed a strong association between T2D and a cluster of *FTO* variants tagged by rs9939609 within intron 1 [25]. Strikingly, this association was abolished after adjusting for BMI, suggesting that the initial association with T2D was mediated by single-nucleotide polymorphism

(SNP)-related effects on BMI. Another study, performed by Froguel et al. [26], employed a different strategy, which aimed at verifying population stratification by testing intergenic regions. The authors described a variant, rs1121980, within intron 1 of *FTO* as strongly associated with early-onset and severe adult obesity. Since then, associations of *FTO* variants have been robustly replicated in numerous GWASs and meta-analyses of GWASs on childhood and adult obesity. *FTO* is ubiquitously expressed in a wide range of organs, so the primary role of *FTO* cannot be postulated directly [27]. Nevertheless, using bioinformatics tools, Gerken et al. [28] showed that murine *Fto* catalyzes the Fe(II)- and 2OG-dependent demethylation of 3-methylthymine in single-stranded DNA, thus suggesting a potential role in nucleic acid demethylation. Subsequent studies indicated the involvement of *FTO* in the regulation of food intake, which was particularly supported by Church et al. [29], who showed that overexpression of *Fto* increased food intake, ultimately resulting in obesity in mice.

Genome-Wide Association Studies and Further Risk Variants beyond FTO

Multiple additional loci associated with obesity have been uncovered in large-scale GWASs and meta-analyses of GWASs conducted within international consortia, such as the Genetic Investigation of ANthropometric Traits (GIANT) consortium [30]. Researchers from the GIANT consortium [30] reported 18 novel loci associated with BMI in a recent large-scale meta-analysis including 249,796 individuals *(RBJ-ADCY3-POMC, GPRC5B-IQCK* (a 21 kb deletion 50 kb away from *GPRC5B*), *MAP2K5-LBXCOR1, QPCTL-GIPR, TNNI3K, SLC39A8, FLJ35779-HMGCR, LRRN6C, TMEM160-ZC3H4, FANCL, CADM2, PRKD1, LRP1B, PTBP2, MTIF3-GTF3A, ZNF608, RPL27A-TUB*, and *NUDT3-HMGA1)*. It is not surprising that some of the genes identified in GWAS, such as *MC4R, POMC, BDNF*, and *SH2B1*, have already been considered as plausible candidate genes for obesity not only due to their function as neuronal regulators of energy balance and food intake but also because they harbor rare variants conferring high obesity risk. It needs to be mentioned, however, that a clear biological link to common obesity is still missing for the majority of loci revealed by GWASs. Furthermore, despite evident advances in the genetics of common obesity, the cumulative risk, allowing prediction of individual obesity risk, is very moderate, and only a small proportion of the heritability of BMI can be explained by the identified variants [31]. Power estimates have suggested hundreds of additional loci with moderate effect sizes to be underpinning common polygenic obesity [30]. This clearly demonstrates the ultimate challenges in genetic research on common obesity and indicates the need for further genetic approaches to be employed in future.

Genome-Wide Association Studies in Children

In contrast to adults, children's phenotypes are less affected by co-morbidities, treatment, and other environmental factors. Furthermore, detailed recording of clinical parameters in the early stages of metabolic alterations is invaluable for understanding the chronology of events ultimately resulting in obesity. For these reasons, children provide a unique tool to uncover genetic factors determining the risk of complex polygenic diseases such as obesity.

Compared with the intensity of genetic research efforts in adults, similar studies in childhood obesity are rather sparse. The few studies in children have been mostly focused on replication of associations observed in adults. For instance, in agreement with findings in adults, variants of *FTO* and *MC4R* have been shown to be associated with obesity in children and adolescents in populations of various ancestries [32–34]. In silico analyses of GWAS data for 25 SNPs in 13 previously reported BMI loci *(NEGR1, SEC16B, TMEM18, INSIG2, SFRS10/ETV5/DGKG, GNPDA2, MTCH2, BDNF, FAIM2, SH2B1, FTO, MC4R*, and *KCTD15)* revealed associations of 15 variants with normalized pediatric BMI data in European Americans, including *FTO* variants [35, 36]. Of note were strong associations of SNPs in *TMEM18, GNDPA2, INSIG2, MC4R, NEGR1, BDNF*, and *KTCD15* with early onset obesity [35]. In particular, the correlation of *INSIG2* variants in children implies that the effects of some genes may be more pronounced in childhood obesity and diminished in later stages of life [37–41]. In contrast, no association in children has been found for *MTCH2* and *SH2B1* variants [35]. Another interesting study assessed the influence of T2D susceptibility variants on BMI in children. One of the previously reported diabetes risk alleles in *HHEX-IDE* was associated with increased BMI in children, which may be in line with the well-established relationship between childhood obesity and T2D in later life [42]. It is also of note that many obesity risk variants in loci such as *FAIM2, NPC1, FTO, MC4R, BDNF*, and *GNPDA2* were related to BMI variation in Chinese children, suggesting that these variants' roles in human obesity are independent of ethnicity [43].

One of the most relevant studies on the genetics of childhood obesity employed a meta-analysis of two GWASs on extreme obesity in French and German children and adolescents [44]. Along with the well-known genetic players such as *FTO, MC4R*, and *TMEM18*, the meta-analysis uncovered two novel loci, *SDCCAG8* and *TNKS/MSRA*, that significantly contributed to variability in body weight. Considering the fact that these two loci have never shown up in meta-analyses of GWASs on obesity in adults, *SDCCAG8* and *TNKS/MSRA* might represent susceptibility loci exclusively influencing childhood obesity. Another recent meta-analysis of GWASs on severe obesity, involving more than 5,000 cases and 8,000 controls, identified two novel loci close to *OLFM4* and *HOXB5* [45]. The study suggested that the role of both genes in obesity is likely to be due to their effects on intestinal function.

Conclusion

Undoubtedly, genetics, in close accord with an unhealthy 'obesogenic' lifestyle in modern societies, has a major influence on an individual's susceptibility to obesity. Despite tremendous success in determining the genetics of common obesity in the last few years, as demonstrated by a number of novel risk loci, only a small proportion of the heritability can be explained so far. Despite a few loci being exclusively associated with early-onset childhood obesity, it has to be acknowledged that most of the major obesity susceptibility genes seem to play a role independent of the respective life stage. In regard to the missing heritability, it seems that the currently accepted common variant-common disease hypothesis might need to be revised and, furthermore, that potential players contributing to common obesity, such as rare and low-frequency variations or epigenetic modifications, need to be considered.

Nevertheless, better knowledge of the genetics of obesity will be fundamental in elucidating the complex etiology of common obesity. This may ultimately lead to novel treatment and prevention strategies, which currently mostly rely on programs targeting weight loss by affecting physical activity and food intake.

Acknowledgments

This work was supported by grants from IFB AdiposityDiseases (ADI-K50D to YB and ADI-K60E to PK) and the German Research Foundation (CRC 1052 to PK; BO 3147/4–14 to YB). IFB AdiposityDiseases is supported by the Federal Ministry of Education and Research (BMBF), Germany, FKZ: 01EO1001. This work was supported by grants from the German Diabetes Association (to YB and PK) and from the DDS Foundation (to YB).

References

1 Must A, Spadano J, Coakley EH, Field AE, Colditz G, et al: The disease burden associated with overweight and obesity. JAMA 1999;282:1523–1529.
2 Kelly T, Yang W, Chen CS, Reynolds K, He J: Global burden of obesity in 2005 and projections to 2030. Int J Obes (Lond) 2008;32:1431–1437.
3 Wang Y, Beydoun MA, Liang L, Caballero B, Kumanyika SK: Will all Americans become overweight or obese? Estimating the progression and cost of the US obesity epidemic. Obesity (Silver Spring) 2008; 16:2323–2330.
4 French SA, Story M, Jeffery RW: Environmental influences on eating and physical activity. Annu Rev-Public. Health 2001;22:309–335.
5 Bell CG, Walley AJ, Froguel P: The genetics of human obesity. Nat Rev Genet 2005;6:221–234.
6 Stunkard AJ, Foch TT, Hrubec Z: A twin study of human obesity. JAMA 1986;256:51–54.
7 Stunkard AJ, Sørensen TI, Hanis C, Teasdale TW, Chakraborty R, et al: An adoption study of human obesity. N Engl J Med 1986;314:193–198.
8 Hinney A, Vogel CI, Hebebrand J: From monogenic to polygenic obesity: recent advances. Eur Child Adolesc Psychiatry 2010;19:297–310.
9 Cheng CY, Kao WH, Patterson N, Tandon A, Haiman CA, et al: Admixture mapping of 15,280 African Americans identifies obesity susceptibility loci on chromosomes 5 and X. PLOS Genet 2009;5: e1000490.
10 Harismendy O, Bansal V, Bhatia G, Nakano M, Scott M, et al: Population sequencing of two endocannabinoid metabolic genes identifies rare and common regulatory variants associated with extreme obesity and metabolite level. Genome Biol 2010;11:R118.
11 Semenkovich CF: Regulation of fatty acid synthase (FAS). Prog Lipid Res 1997;36:43–53.
12 Mobbs CV, Makimura H: Block the FAS, lose the fat. Nat Med 2002;8:335–336.
13 Kovacs P, Harper I, Hanson RL, Infante AM, Bogardus C, et al: A novel missense substitution (Val1483Ile) in the fatty acid synthase gene (FAS) is associated with percentage of body fat and substrate oxidation rates in nondiabetic Pima Indians. Diabetes 2004;53:1915–1919.
14 Körner A, Ma L, Franks PW, Kiess W, Baier LJ, et al: Sex-specific effect of the Val1483Ile polymorphism in the fatty acid synthase gene (FAS) on body mass index and lipid profile in Caucasian children. Int J Obes (Lond) 2007;31:353–358.

15 Berndt J, Kovacs P, Ruschke K, Klöting N, Fasshauer M, et al: Fatty acid synthase gene expression in human adipose tissue: association with obesity and type 2 diabetes. Diabetologia 2007;50:1472–1480.
16 Schleinitz D, Klöting N, Körner A, Berndt J, Reichenbächer M, et al: Effect of genetic variation in the human fatty acid synthase gene (FASN) on obesity and fat depot-specific mRNA expression. Obesity (Silver Spring) 2010;18:1218–1225.
17 Meyre D, Lecoeur C, Delplanque J, Francke S, Vatin V, et al: A genome-wide scan for childhood obesity-associated traits in French families shows significant linkage on chromosome 6q22.31-q23.2. Diabetes 2004;53:803–811.
18 Maddux BA, Goldfine ID: Membrane glycoprotein PC-1 inhibition of insulin receptor function occurs via direct interaction with the receptor alpha-subunit. Diabetes 2000;49:13–19.
19 Pizzuti A, Frittitta L, Argiolas A, Baratta R, Goldfine ID, et al: A polymorphism (K121Q) of the human glycoprotein PC-1 gene coding region is strongly associated with insulin resistance. Diabetes 1999;48:1881–1884.
20 Bochenski J, Placha G, Wanic K, Malecki M, Sieradzki J, et al: New polymorphism of ENPP1 (PC-1) is associated with increased risk of type 2 diabetes among obese individuals. Diabetes 2006;55:2626–2630.
21 Abate N, Chandalia M, Satija P, Adams-Huet B, Grundy SM, et al: ENPP1/PC-1 K121Q polymorphism and genetic susceptibility to type 2 diabetes. Diabetes 2005;54:1207–1213.
22 Meyre D, Bouatia-Naji N, Tounian A, Samson C, Lecoeur C, et al: Variants of ENPP1 are associated with childhood and adult obesity and increase the risk of glucose intolerance and type 2 diabetes. Nat Genet 2005;37:863–867.
23 Böttcher Y, Körner A, Reinehr T, Enigk B, Kiess W, et al: ENPP1 variants and haplotypes predispose to early onset obesity and impaired glucose and insulin metabolism in German obese children. J Clin Endocrinol Metab 2006;91:4948–4952.
24 Wang R, Zhou D, Xi B, Ge X, Zhu P, et al: ENPP1/PC-1 Gene K121Q polymorphism is associated with obesity in European adult populations: evidence from a meta-analysis involving 24,324 subjects. Biomed Environ Sci 2011;24:200–206.
25 Frayling TM, Timpson NJ, Weedon MN, Zeggini E, Freathy RM, et al: A common variant in the FTO gene is associated with body mass index and predisposes to childhood and adult obesity. Science 2007;316:889–894.
26 Dina C, Meyre D, Gallina S, Durand E, Körner A, et al: Variation in FTO contributes to childhood obesity and severe adult obesity. Nat Genet 2007;39:724–726.
27 Stratigopoulos G, Leibel RL: FTO gains function. Nat Genet 2010;42:1038–1039.
28 Gerken T, Girard CA, Tung YC, Webby CJ, Saudek V, et al: The obesity-associated FTO gene encodes a 2-oxoglutarate-dependent nucleic acid demethylase. Science 2007;318:1469–1472.
29 Church C, Moir L, McMurray F, Girard C, Banks GT, et al: Overexpression of Fto leads to increased food intake and results in obesity. Nat Genet 2010;42:1086–1092.
30 Speliotes EK, Willer CJ, Berndt SI, Monda KL, Thorleifsson G, et al: Association analyses of 249,796 individuals reveal 18 new loci associated with body mass index. Nat Genet 2010;42:937–948.
31 Manolio TA, Collins FS, Cox NJ, Goldstein DB, Hindorff LA, et al: Finding the missing heritability of complex diseases. Nature 2009;461:747–753.
32 den Hoed M, Ekelund U, Brage S, Grontved A, Zhao JH, et al: Genetic susceptibility to obesity and related traits in childhood and adolescence: influence of loci identified by genome-wide association studies. Diabetes 2010;59:2980–2988.
33 Liu G, Zhu H, Lagou V, Gutin B, Stallmann-Jorgensen IS, et al: FTO variant rs9939609 is associated with body mass index and waist circumference, but not with energy intake or physical activity in European- and African-American youth. BMC Med Genet 2010;11:57.
34 Xi B, Shen Y, Zhang M, Liu X, Zhao X, et al: The common rs9939609 variant of the fat mass and obesity-associated gene is associated with obesity risk in children and adolescents of Beijing, China. BMC. Med Genet 2010;11:107.
35 Zhao J, Bradfield JP, Li M, Wang K, Zhang H, et al: The role of obesity-associated loci identified in genome-wide association studies in the determination of pediatric BMI. Obesity (Silver Spring) 2009;17:2254–2257.
36 Zhao J, Grant SFA: Genetics of childhood obesity. J Obes 2011;2011:845148.
37 Bressler J, Fornage M, Hanis CL, Kao WH, Lewis CE, et al: The INSIG2 rs7566605 genetic variant does not play a major role in obesity in a sample of 24,722 individuals from four cohorts. BMC Med Genet 2009;10:56.
38 Campa D, Hüsing A, McKay JD, Sinilnikova O, Vogel U, et al: The INSIG2 rs7566605 polymorphism is not associated with body mass index and breast cancer risk. BMC Cancer 2010;10:563.
39 Deka RL, Pal P, Toelupe PT, Laumoli TS, Xi H, et al: A tagging SNP in INSIG2 is associated with obesity-related phenotypes among Samoans. BMC Med Genet 2009;10:143.

40 Heid IM, Huth C, Loos RJ, Kronenberg F, Adamkova V, et al: Meta-analysis of the INSIG2 association with obesity including 74,345 individuals: does heterogeneity of estimates relate to study design? PLoS Genet 2009;5:e1000694.
41 Herbert A, Gerry NP, McQueen MB, Heid IM, Pfeufer A, et al: A common genetic variant is associated with adult and childhood obesity. Science 2006; 312:279–283.
42 Zhao J, Bradfield JP, Zhang H, Annaiah K, Wang K, et al: Examination of all type 2 diabetes GWAS loci reveals HHEX-IDE as a locus influencing pediatric BMI. Diabetes 2010;59:751–755.
43 Wu L, Xi B, Zhang M, Shen Y, Zhao X, et al: Associations of six single nucleotide polymorphisms in obesity-related genes with BMI and risk of obesity in Chinese children. Diabetes 2010;59:3085–3089.
44 Scherag A, Dina C, Hinney A, Vatin V, Scherag S, et al: Two new loci for body-weight regulation identified in a joint analysis of genome-wide association studies for early-onset extreme obesity in French and German study groups. PLoS Genet 2010;6:e1000916.
45 Bradfield JP, Taal HR, Timpson NJ, Scherag A, Lecoeur C, et al: A genome-wide association meta-analysis identifies new childhood obesity loci. Nat Genet 2012;44:526–531.

Peter Kovacs, PhD
IFB AdiposityDiseases, Medical Faculty, University of Leipzig
Liebigstrasse 21
DE–04103 Leipzig (Germany)
E-Mail peter.kovacs@medizin.uni-leipzig.de

Kiess W, Wabitsch M, Maffeis C, Sharma AM (eds): Metabolic Syndrome and Obesity in Childhood and Adolescence. Pediatr Adolesc Med. Basel, Karger, 2015, vol 19, pp 40–52 (DOI: 10.1159/000368105)

Nutrition

Hermann Kalhoff[a] · Mathilde Kersting[b]

[a]Paediatric Clinic, Dortmund, and [b]Research Institute of Child Nutrition, University of Bonn, Bonn, Germany

Abstract

The rapid increase in obesity prevalence during the past decades points to the important impact of environmental changes on the development of overweight in children and adolescents. A mismatch between increasing energy consumption in an attractive and abundant food environment and decreasing physical activity with the adoption of a more sedentary lifestyle is the key factor underlying constant increases in body mass index. Considering the effect of energy imbalance on body weight, a small but persistent average daily imbalance between intake and expenditure is sufficient to explain the weight gain observed during the development of overweight and obesity, and the influences of nutrition on the development of these conditions vary according to life stage and circumstance. Parental dietary intake and familial nutritional behaviour are important components in the development of childhood nutritional habits. We discuss the possible contributions of several nutritional factors to the antenatal and postnatal environments and the impacts of nutrition during infancy, childhood and adolescence. However, nutrition involves a complex interplay among dietary behaviour, food selection and nutrient supply that complicates the aetiological analysis of the development of adiposity. In particular, a diet comprising foods with high energy densities may be a key factor that increases the risk of developing overweight during childhood and adolescence. The establishment of an optimised mixed diet may serve as a guideline to evaluate and further improve dietary intake in the family setting and in the catering industry, thus reducing the nutritional causes of the development of obesity and metabolic syndrome.

Introduction

The worldwide prevalence of childhood obesity has risen greatly over the last 3 decades, causing a wide range of serious medical complaints and increasing the risk of premature morbidity and death later in life. In spite of recent reports suggesting a levelling off of the obesity epidemic in some countries, the societal burden of paediatric obesity is still high [1–5].

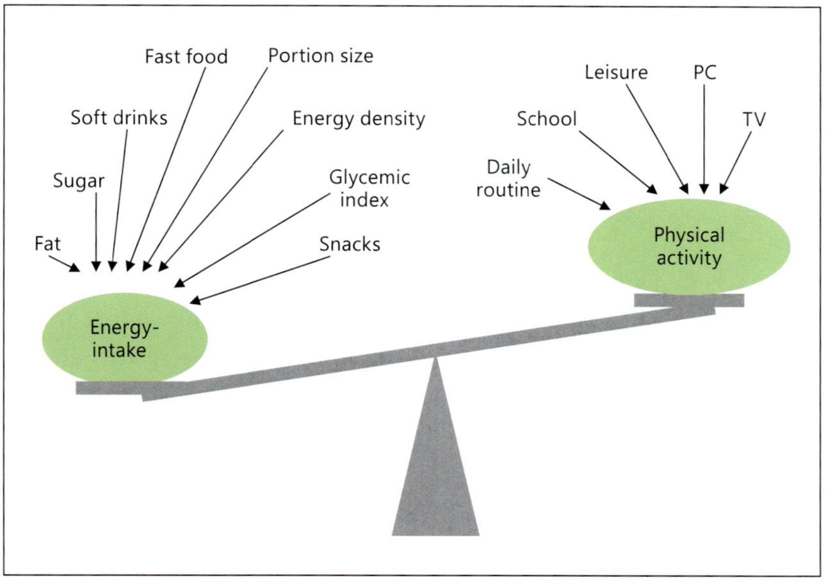

Fig. 1. Components of dietary energy intake and energy expenditure that may impact the development of overweight and obesity in children and adolescents.

Because obese children tend to become obese adults and are at increased risk of several acute and chronic diseases, such as hypertension, dyslipidaemia, coronary heart disease, cancer, gout, psychosocial disability and musculoskeletal disorders, the prevention of obesity must start in childhood at the latest [6, 7].

Weight control during development is balanced between overall energy intake and energy expenditure and is mainly achieved by physical activity (fig. 1). Children must sustain a careful balance between energy consumption and expenditure to maintain their individual (recommended) body weight and to assure adequate growth.

A tiny daily energy gap that is constant and longstanding usually causes individuals to become overweight because it can add up to considerable gains in body weight over a number of years [8, 9]. Longitudinal data included in the Kiel Obesity Prevention Study were used to calculate energy gain in normal-weight children who maintained their weight or became overweight and ranged in age from 6–10 and 10–14 years. The mean energy gains (kcal/day) of these two age groups were approximately 25 kcal for the children aged 6 to 10 and approximately 40 kcal/d for those aged 10 to 14 [10]. Thus, halting the progression of obesity would require a comparably small but regular decrease in daily energy intake, ideally combined with a tiny increase in daily physical energy expenditure [11].

The focus of this article is to assess the role of dietary factors and food habits in contributing to the development of obesity during early life, childhood and adolescence [8, 9].

Nutrition and Obesity – According to Developmental Stages

Nutritional influences on the development of overweight and obesity vary by life stage and circumstance. In the following section, we discuss important relevant aspects structured according to infant and child development.

Antenatal

The antenatal environment has an important impact on foetal development via influences such as antenatal stress, placental function and maternal nutrition. Some effects seem to persist into adulthood, increasing the likelihood for obesity-related conditions, such as the development of metabolic syndrome [12].

Maternal overweight before and high weight gain during pregnancy are positively linked to child overweight and obesity. The odds of having an obese child increase with every kilogram of weight gained during pregnancy [13–15].

Maternal malnutrition during the first 2 trimesters of pregnancy is linked to an increased risk of obesity and the development of metabolic syndrome in young children [16]. This may be due to structural and functional abnormalities of endocrine system development due to nutrient restriction and disturbances in glucose and insulin homeostasis during pregnancy.

Infancy and Early Childhood

Early childhood feeding seems to be a major contributor to childhood obesity. Both the type of infant feeding (e.g. breast milk versus formula) and the rate of weight gain during infancy are linked to weight status in later childhood in addition to cardiovascular risk factors [17, 18]. A recent study that analysed data obtained from a nationally representative database has revealed that early excess weight gain is a key predictor of obesity in school children from kindergarten through the eighth grade [4].

During infancy, dietary intake may have greater impacts on nutrient balance and hormone responses than energy expenditure. A large prospective cohort study has shown that dietary energy intake during infancy determines infant weight gain and seems to influence the risk of childhood obesity. These results could be demonstrated at least among formula- and mixed-fed infants [19].

Breastfeeding: Breast milk is unequivocally recommended as the exclusive nutrition source during the first 4–6 months of life. However, regarding the later development of obesity, there is only moderate evidence for a protective effect of breastfeeding. In some studies, breastfeeding has been found to lower the risk of the development of obesity during childhood [17, 20] (for a review, see [21]). Recent analysis has indicated that breastfeeding has long-term favourable effects on adult body composition, extremes of adiposity and insulin metabolism; however, these effects were only observed in women [22]. By contrast, high protein intake from formula in infants seems to be associated with a higher body mass index, which lasts until the child is 6 years of age [23].

Introduction of Solid Food: The delayed introduction of solid food has been suggested to reduce the odds of overweight in children [24]; however, a literature review could not verify this association [25]. Thus, the available evidence so far has not provided sufficient information to clarify this issue.

In healthy, term, appropriate-for-gestational age children, a consistently high fat intake during the second year of life modifies the subsequent effects of rapid weight gain on the longitudinal development of fat mass, thus inhibiting its normal physiologic decrease, resulting in a larger body fat percentage [26].

Taken together, systematic analysis of thirty prospective studies has identified strong independent associations of childhood overweight with maternal overweight during pregnancy, high infant birth weight and rapid weight gain during the first year of life. A meta-analysis comparing breastfed with non-breastfed infants has found a slight decrease in the odds of overweight due to breastfeeding. Moreover, there is some evidence associating the early introduction of solid food with overweight [27].

Childhood and Adolescence

Fruits and Vegetables: Eating a diet high in fruits and vegetables may help to reduce body weight and fat accretion. Fruits and vegetables have high water and high dietary fibre contents, making them low in energy density [28]. Thus, they help to reduce total energy intake by displacing energy-dense food from the diet. Moreover, the reduction in the glycaemic load of food alters postprandial hormones and could be involved in initiating satiety [29]. Whereas this inverse relationship between the intake of vegetables and fruits and adiposity has not been observed in all studies [30, 31], no studies have shown a worsening of child weight status in association with increases in vegetable and fruit consumption.

Energetic Beverages: Children and adolescents derive approximately 20% of their energy intake from added sugars in food items and beverages [32]. These sugar-sweetened foods seem to strongly contribute to increased body mass index in children [33–36].

The long-term high consumption of sugar-sweetened beverages has been suggested to be associated with high body weight in adolescents, especially in girls [37]. Compared with research in the US and elsewhere, the levels of sweetened milk and fruit juice intake are unique for European adolescents. A survey has reported that European adolescents consume an average of 1,455 ml/day of beverages, with water being consumed by the largest proportion of these individuals and at the greatest volume. In this study, beverages provided 1,609 kJ/day, of which 30.4, 20.7, and 18.1% came from sugar-sweetened beverages, sweetened milk, and fruit juice, respectively [38]. The epidemiological evidence that drinks containing added sugars, including sucrose and high-fructose corn syrup, are a cause of overweight and obesity is consistent [36]. However, there is no unequivocal consensus on the strength of the evidence for causality [39].

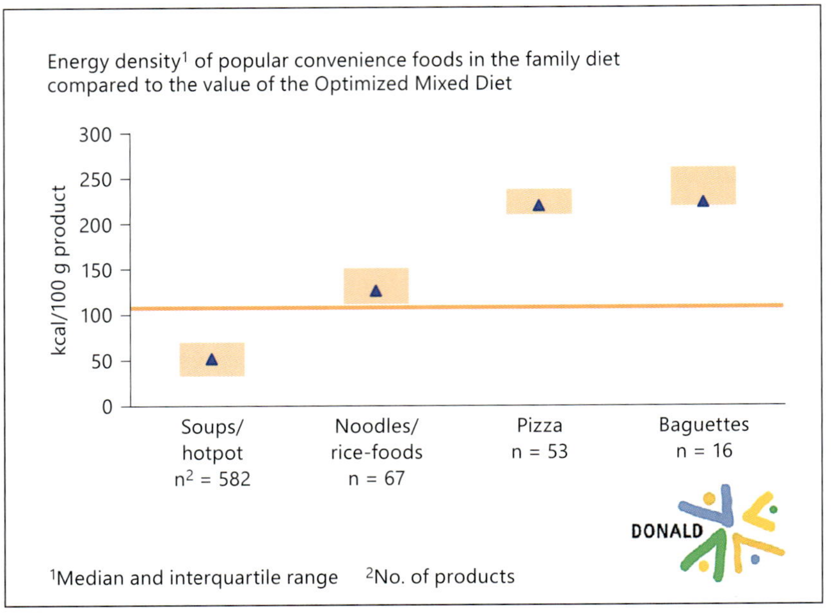

Fig. 2. Energy densities (median and interquartile range) of popular convenience foods consumed in family diets compared to those of foods consumed in the optimised mixed diet.

Food and Eating Environment

Family: Home environment and family feeding behaviours play important roles in the development of childhood nutritional habits. The parental intake of vegetables and fruits, for example, is positively associated with the consumption of these foods in their children [40]. General parenting and parental feeding practices have strong impacts on the evolution of child food intake and on the development of obesity [41, 42]. In general, parents may be advised to encourage moderation rather than overconsumption and to emphasise healthful food choices rather than restrictive eating patterns [43].

Eating Frequency: Meta-analysis of original observational studies has shown that higher eating frequency is associated with lower body weight during childhood and adolescence, especially in males [44]. This is in line with observations showing more favourable nutrient intake profiles and adiposity indices in children/adolescents who eat breakfast compared to those who skip this meal [45].

Convenience Food: In developed countries, pre-prepared commercial foods (convenience foods) are one aspect of modern dietary habits. Data from the Dortmund Nutritional and Anthropometric Longitudinally Designed Study have shown that convenience food is characterised by high fat content and high numbers of flavourings and food additives [46]. Further analysis has shown a significant negative correlation between nutrient quality index and the increased consumption of convenience foods (fig. 2) [47].

Along with energy-dense convenience food, such as French fries, hamburgers, salty snacks, pizzas and sugared drinks, portion size has increased over the years [48]. This amounts to an increased risk of obesity because portion size seems to be the primary determinant of energy intake, more so than energy density [49]. Generally, it seems to be good advice to base diets on fresh and minimally processed foods if possible [50].

Food Marketing: Given the reduction in physical activity and specific food manufacturing and marketing practices, such as vending machines in schools, the increased availability of food may be another key factor explaining the obesity epidemic [51]. Moreover, in many developed countries, foods with high energy densities are relatively cheap. Therefore, economic constraints might favour the consumption of high-energy dense food in low-income groups, thus contributing to their excessive nutritional energy intake [52]. Environmental-level interventions, such as reducing food advertisements targeting young children, increasing the availability of smaller portions and providing alternatives to sugar-sweetened soft drinks would encourage individual and family-level behavioural changes, thus supporting the prevention of obesity [53].

It has been shown that a combined environmental and educational intervention strategy with a single focus on the promotion and provision of drinking water might be an effective tool in the prevention of childhood overweight [54].

But: Nutrition Is Complex

Problems with nutritional analysis start with methodological limitations in dietary intake assessment and extend to questioning the interrelationships between energy-yielding nutrients and their respective foods that exist during the development of overweight and obesity.

Underreporting seems to be a relevant issue in the self-assessment of caloric intake by obese subjects. Therefore, the plausibility of self-reported food intake data is of special importance [55].

Randomised controlled trials performed in population settings are rare. Arguments for the effects of several subcomponents of nutrition on the development of overweight and obesity thus tend to rely on associations between the putative factors and the obesity rate derived from a complex group of children and adolescents. These considerations do not disprove the importance of the nutritional causes that have been reported but do highlight their sometimes less-than-unequivocal evidential basis.

Moreover, there is some consensus that in people on *ad libitum* diets, the body fat changes that occur along with intake modification seem to be mediated via these alterations in energy intake [34, 36].

A Prominent Role of Energy Density of Food

One key factor underlying the nutritional causes of childhood overweight and obesity may be the energy density of food, which is defined as the energy content (in kcal of kJ) per unit weight (e.g. g or 100 g). High energy-dense foods, particularly sugary drinks and 'fast foods', are probably a cause of weight gain, over-

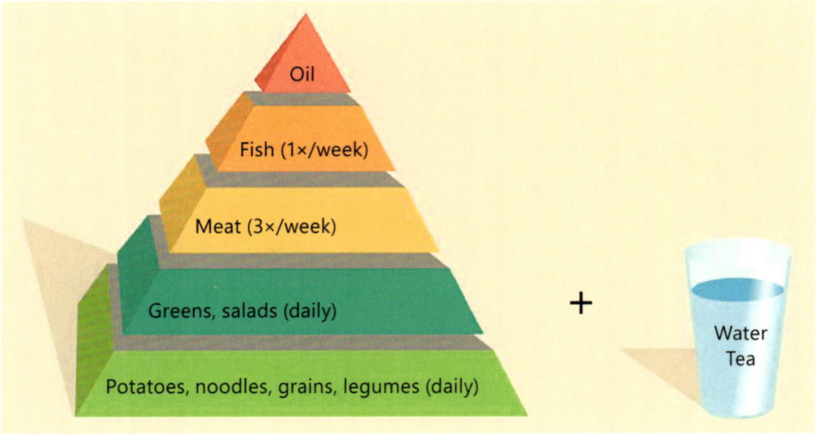

Fig. 3. Optimised meal composition including foods with low energy densities for consumption by children and adolescents.

weight and obesity [56]. Such foods are typically high in fats and/or sugars, contain little water or dietary fibre and are often low in micronutrients. By contrast, low energy-dense foods, typically foods that are high in fibre and are bulky because of their water content, are probably protective against overweight and obesity. Such foods include vegetables and fruits, cereals (whole grain) and pulses (legumes). They are often micronutrient-dense, meaning that they are high in vitamins, minerals, and other bioactive compounds (fig. 3).

The Dietary Guidelines for Americans encourage the consumption of food that is low in energy density. Such an eating pattern is characterised by a relatively high intake of vegetables, fruits, and dietary fibre and a relatively low intake of total fat, saturated fat, and added sugar [57, 58]. Given that numerous studies have shown that energy density is one important factor influencing increases in body weight, the German Nutritional Society has recently introduced energy density as a useful concept in the evaluation of foods. The rationale is that a nutritional regimen including low energy-dense foods can help to maintain or reduce body weight in children and adolescents as well as in adults [59].

Dietary Fibre Intake: The energy density of food can be reduced by an increase in dietary fibre consumption in children. A recent review has summarised currently existing evidence pertaining to the implications of dietary fibre intake on constipation, obesity and diabetes in children. The authors have concluded that the known health benefits justify an increased awareness of dietary fibre intake in children [60].

Water: Increasing dietary water intake is another potential way to reduce energy that theoretically not only increases the volume of food but also lowers the intake of sweetened beverages in favour of plain water. Whereas studies of individuals dieting for weight loss or maintenance have suggested the weight-reducing effect of increased water consumption, studies in general mixed-weight populations thus far have

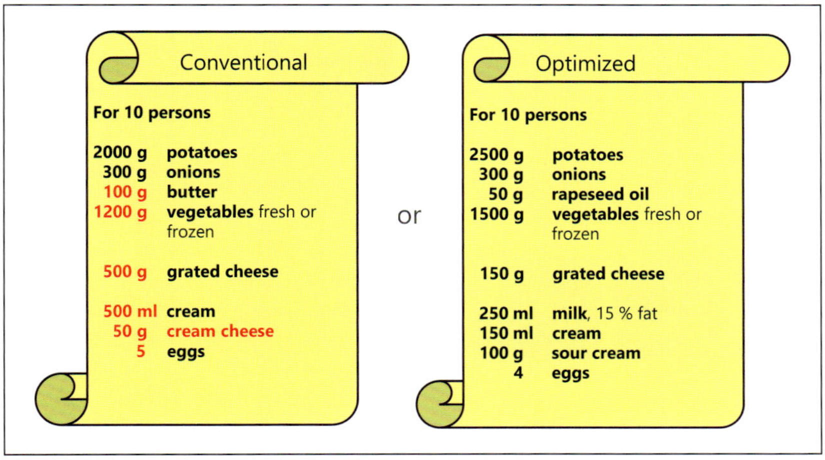

Fig. 4. Decreasing energy densities by cautious exchange of high-fat with low-fat components (recipe).

yielded inconsistent results. Therefore, in real-life studies, the association between water intake and reduced daily energy intake via food has remained low, mostly because of the lack of good-quality studies [61].

Evaluation of a Given Diet

Dietary patterns are relevant to the development of overweight and obesity, not only during infancy but also during childhood (at the beginning and during the course of primary school) and young adulthood [38, 62]. During infancy, we recommend feeding for the first year according to the food-based dietary guidelines of ESPGHAN in Germany [63]. The guidelines include exclusive breastfeeding during the first 4–6 months of life and the introduction of increasing proportions of complementary foods during the second 6 months, including some vegetables and fruits [63, 64].

Regarding children and adolescents, in 2011, the ESPGHAN Committee on Nutrition published a commentary aimed at providing a summary of the role of nutrition-related factors on obesity prevention in children aged 2–18 years. Experts recommend the preferential intake of slow-absorbing carbohydrates, the use of plant-based foods as the main dietary constituents and the use of plain water as the main source of fluids. They also recommend that children eat at least 4 meals a day, starting with breakfast. Regular family meals are encouraged, whereas the regular consumption of fast food is discouraged [65].

In line with these recommendations, we propose an optimised mixed-diet concept that is easy to adopt in the family setting and in the catering industry (fig. 4). This concept translates scientific nutrient-related recommendations into food- and meal-

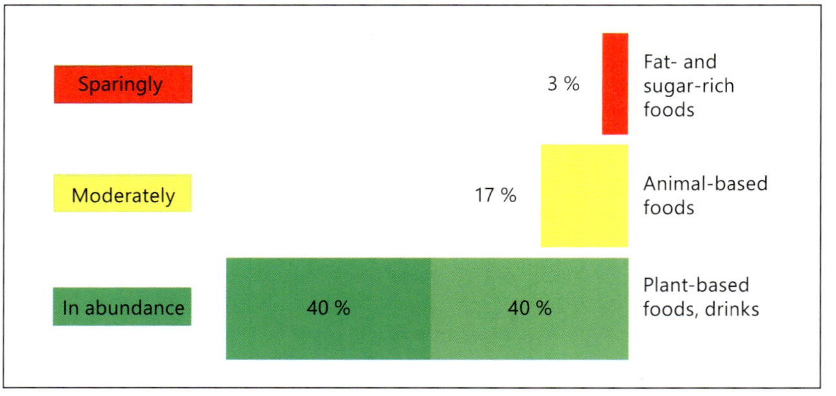

Fig. 5. Subsuming food-based dietary guidelines into 3 main rules for food selection in a balanced diet for children and adolescents.

Table 1. Exchanging high- with low-energy density foods

Portion	kcal	Portion	kcal
Salami, 30 g	115	Boiled ham, 30 g	40
Nut-nougat cream, 20 g	105	Marmalade, honey, 20 g	55
Potato chips, 50 g	270	Salt sticks, 50 g	165
Cheesecake, 100 g	230	Apple pie (yeast dough), 100 g	140
1 Croissant, 45 g	185	1 Raisin roll, 45 g	120
1 Chocolate bar, 40 g	200	Fruit gum, 40 g	130
1 Cream ice	290	1 Calippo water ice	100
1 Glass (full-cream) milk	160	1 Glass buttermilk	95

Table 2. Reducing energy density while maintaining recipe quality

Conventional recipe	Optimised recipe
1 L Milk, 3.5% cream	1 L Milk 1.5% cream
2 Packages chocolate pudding powder	2 Packages chocolate pudding powder
6 Tablespoons sugar	3 Tablespoons sugar
2 Tbsp. whipped cream, 30% fat	1 Cup yoghurt (500 g)
4 Fresh pears, steamed (200 g)	6 Fresh pears, steamed (300 g)
16 g fat and 292 kcal per portion	2.2 g fat and 150 kcal per portion

based dietary guidelines. The food options can be summarised with three simple rules as follows: plant-based foods and drinks should be consumed in abundance, animal-based foods in moderation and fat and sugar-rich foods sparingly (fig. 5) [66].

The EFSA Panel on Dietetic Products, Nutrition and Allergies [67] has recommended this total-diet concept as an example for the establishment of food-based

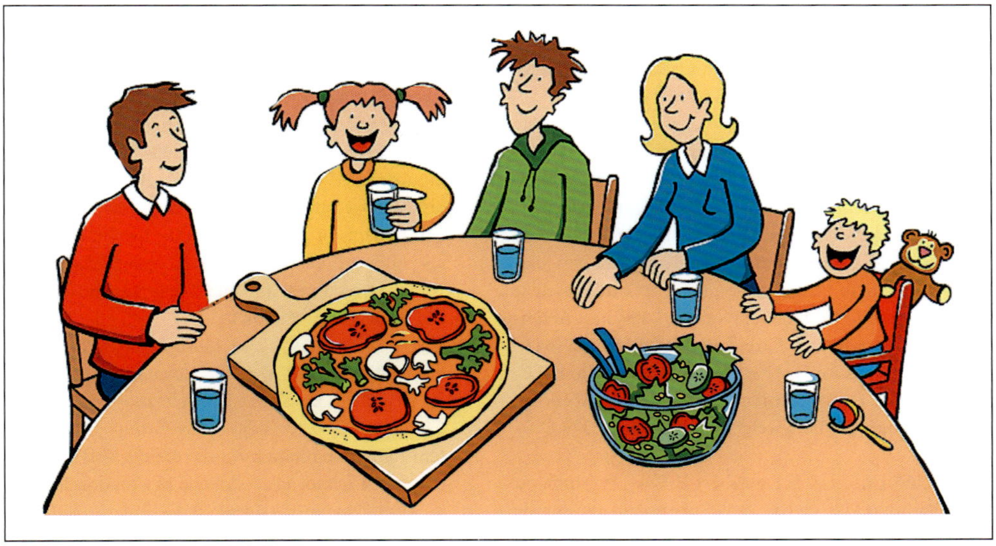

Fig. 6. Example of a healthy meal comprising optimised convenience food.

dietary guidelines for children and adolescents aged 1 to 18 years. This optimised mixed diet concept (e.g. tables 1, 2) has recently been utilised to establish a healthy diet regimen in a paediatric hospital, for which five meals a day were planned for children, including two cold principal meals, one hot principal meal and two snacks [68].

Considering other environmental factors associated with childhood obesity risk, such as parental overweight and socioeconomic status, future interventions should give specific attention to children from overweight and/or low socioeconomic status parents [69].

In summary, key recommendations for healthy diets in children and adolescents allow for the avoidance of the potential causes of overweight and obesity by communicating positive messages with regard to preferring foods with low energy densities, consuming 4–5 regular meals a day (starting with breakfast), avoiding big portion sizes, increasing fluid intake (preferably plain water) and encouraging family meals (fig. 6).

References

1 Han JC, Lawlor DA, Kimm SYS: Childhood obesity. Lancet 2010;375:1737–1748.
2 Brüne M, Hochberg Z: Secular trends in new childhood epidemics: insights from evolutionary medicine. BMC Med 2013;11:226.
3 Slimming down childhood obesity. Editorial. Lancet 2013;382:572.
4 Cunningham SA, Kramer MR, Narayan KM: Incidence of childhood obesity in the United States. N Engl J Med 2014;370:403–411.
5 Wabitsch M, Moss A, Kromeyer-Hauschild K: Unexpected plateauing of childhood obesity rates in developed countries. BMC Med 2014;12:17.
6 Rauh-Pfeiffer A, Koletzko B: Overweight and obesity in childhood and adolescence. Monatsschr Kinderheilkd 2007;155:469–483.

7 Muckelbauer R, Kalhoff H, Müller-Nordhorn J, Kersting M: Childhood overweight and obesity: introduction into epidemiology and prevention strategies. Curr. Nutr Food Sc 2011;7:191–199.

8 Steinberger J, Daniels SR, Eckel RH, Hayman L, Lustig RH, et al: Progress and challenges in metabolic syndrome in children and adolescents: a scientific statement from the American Heart Association Atherosclerosis, Hypertension, and Obesity in the Young Committee of the Council on Cardiovascular Disease in the Young; Council on Cardiovascular Nursing; and Council on Nutrition, Physical Activity, and Metabolism. Circulation 2009;119:628–647.

9 Hall KD, Sacks G, Chandramohan D, Chow CC, Wang YC, et al: Quantification of the effect of energy imbalance on bodyweight. Lancet 2011;378:826–837.

10 Plachta-Danielzik S, Landsberg B, Bosy-Westphal A, Johannsen M, Lange D, et al: Energy gain and energy gap in normal-weight children: longitudinal data of the KOPS. Obesity (Silver Spring) 2008;16:777–783.

11 Hill JO, Wyatt HR, Peters JC: Energy balance and obesity. Circulation 2012;126:126–132.

12 Barker DJ, Eriksson JG, Forsén T, Osmond C: Fetal origins of adult disease: strength of effects and biological basis. Int J Epidemiol 2002;31:1235–1239.

13 Cho NH, Silverman BL, Rizzo TA, Metzger BE: Correlations between the intrauterine metabolic environment and blood pressure in adolescent offspring of diabetic mothers. J Pediatr 2000;136:587–592.

14 Wrotniak BH, Shults J, Butts S, Stettler N: Gestational weight gain and risk of overweight in the offspring at age 7 y in a multicenter, multiethnic cohort study. Am J Clin Nutr 2008;87:1818–1824.

15 Latouche C, Heywood SE, Henry SL, Ziemann M, Lazarus R, et al: Maternal overnutrition programs changes in the expression of skeletal muscle genes that are associated with insulin resistance and defects of oxidative phosphorylation in adult male rat offspring. J Nutr 2014;144:237–244.

16 Armitage JA, Khan IY, Taylor PD, Nathanielsz PW, Poston L: Developmental programming of the metabolic syndrome by maternal nutritional imbalance: how strong is the evidence from experimental models in mammals? J Physiol 2004;561:355–377.

17 von Kries R, Koletzko B, Sauerwald T, von Mutius E, Barnert D, et al: Breast feeding and obesity: cross sectional study. BMJ 1999;319:147–150.

18 Stettler N, Zemel BS, Kumanyika S, Stallings VA: Infant weight gain and childhood overweight status in a multicenter, cohort study. Pediatr 2002;109:194–199.

19 Ong KK, Emmett PM, Noble S, Ness A, Dunger DB, et al: Dietary energy intake at the age of 4 months predicts postnatal weight gain and childhood body mass index. Pediatrics 2006;117:e503–e508.

20 Armstrong J, Reilly JJ, Child Health Information Team: Breastfeeding and lowering the risk of childhood obesity. Lancet 2002;359:2003–2004.

21 Arenz S, Rückerl R, Koletzko B, von Kries R: Breastfeeding and childhood obesity – a systematic review. Int J Obes Relat Metab Disord 2004;28:1247–1256.

22 Günther A, Walz H, Kroke A, Wudy SA, Riedel C, et al: Breastfeeding and its prospective association with components of the GH-IGF-Axis, insulin resistance and body adiposity measures in young adulthood – insights from linear and quantile regression analysis. PLOS ONE 2013;8:e79436.

23 Weber M, Grote V, Closa-Monasterolo R, Escribano J, Langhendries JP, Dain E, Giovannini M, Verduci E, Gruszfeld D, Socha P, Koletzko B, European Childhood Obesity Trial Study Group: Lower protein content in infant formula reduces BMI and obesity risk at school age: follow up of a randomized trial. Am J Clin Nutr 2014;99:1041–1051.

24 Seach KA, Dharmage SC, Lowe AJ, Dixon JB: Delayed introduction of solid feeding. Int J Obes 2010; 34:1475–1479.

25 Yew KS, Webber B, Hodges J, Carter NJ: Clinical inquiries: are there any known health risks to early introduction of solids to an infant's diet? J Fam Pract 2009;58:219–220.

26 Karaolis-Danckert N, Günther AL, Kroke A, Hornberg C, Buyken AE: How early dietary factors modify the effect of rapid weight gain in infancy on subsequent body-composition development in term children whose birth weight was appropriate for gestational age. Am J Clin Nutr 2007;86:1700–1708.

27 Weng SF, Redsell SA, Swift JA, Yang M, Glazebrook CP: Systematic review and meta-analyses of risk factors for childhood overweight identifiable during infancy. Arch Dis Child 2012;97:1019–1026.

28 Fisher JO, Arreoala A, Birch LL, Rolls BJ: Portion size effects on daily energy intake in low-income Hispanic and African American children and their mothers. Am J Clin Nutr 2007;86:174–179.

29 Livesay G, Taylor R, Hulshof T, Howlett J: Glycemic response and health-a systematic review and meta-analysis: relations between dietary glycemic properties and health outcomes. Am J Clin Nutr 2008;87: 258–268.

30 Yannakoulia M, Ntalla I, Papoutsakis C, Farmaki AE, Dedoussis GV: Consumption of vegetables, cooked meals, and eating dinner is negatively associated with overweight status in children. J Pediatr 2010;157:815–820.

31 Newby PK: Plant foods and plant-based diets: protective against childhood obesity? Am J Clin Nutr 2009;89:1572S–1587S.

32 Reedy J, Krebs-Smith SM: Dietary sources of energy, solid fats, and added sugars among children and adolescents in the United States. J AM DIET Assoc 2010;110:1477–1484.

33 Malik VS, Schulze MB, Hu FB: Intake of sugar-sweetened beverages and weight gain: a systematic review. Am J Clin Nutr 2006;84:274–288.
34 Moreno LA, Rodríguez G: Dietary risk factors for development of childhood obesity. Curr Opin Clin Nutr Metab Care 2007;10:336–341.
35 Lanfer A, Hebestreit A, Ahrens W: Diet and eating habits in relation to the development of obesity in children and adolescents. Bundesgesundheitsblatt Gesundheitsforschung Gesundheitsschutz 2010;53: 690–698.
36 Morenga LT, Mallard S, Mann J: Dietary sugars and body weight: systematic review and meta-analyses of randomised controlled trials and cohort studies. BMJ 2012;345:e7492.
37 Libuda L, Alexy U, Sichert-Hellert W, Stehle P, Karaolis-Danckert N, et al: Pattern of beverage consumption and long-term association with body-weight status in German adolescents—results from the DONALD study. Br J Nutr 2008;99:1370–1379.
38 Duffey KJ, Huybrechts I, Mouratidou T, Libuda L, Kersting M, et al: Beverage consumption among European adolescents in the HELENA study. Eur J Clin Nutr 2012;66:244–252.
39 Massougbodji J, Le Bodo Y, Fratu R, De Wals P: Reviews examining sugar-sweetened beverages and body weight: correlates of their quality and conclusions. Am J Clin Nutr 2014;99:1096–1104.
40 Vereecken C, Rovner A, Maes L: Associations of parenting styles, parental feeding practices and child characteristics with young children's fruit and vegetable consumption. Appetite 2010;55:589–596.
41 Rhee KE, Lumeng JC, Appugliese DP, Kaciroti N, Bradley RH: Parenting styles and overweight status in the first grade. Pediatr 2006;117:2047–2054.
42 Sleddens EF, Gerards SM, Thijs C, de Vries NK, Kremers SP: General parenting, childhood overweight and obesity-inducing behaviors: a review. Int J Pediatr Obes 2011;6:e12–e27.
43 Loth KA, MacLehose RF, Fulkerson JA, Crow S, Neumark-Sztainer D: Food-related parenting practices and adolescent weight status: a population-based study. Pediatrics 2013;131:e1443–e1450.
44 Kaisari P, Yannakoulia M, Panagiotakos DB: Eating frequency and overweight and obesity in children and adolescents: a meta-analysis. Pediatrics 2013; 131:958–967.
45 Deshmukh-Taskar PR, Nicklas TA, O'Neil CE, Keast DR, Radcliffe JD, et al: The relationship of breakfast skipping and type of breakfast consumption with nutrient intake and weight status in children and adolescents: the national health and nutrition examination survey 1999–2006. J AM DIET Assoc 2010;110: 869–878.
46 Alexy U, Sichert-Hellert W, Rode T, Kersting M: Convenience food in the diet of children and adolescents: consumption and composition. Br J Nutr 2008;99:345–351.
47 Alexy U, Libuda L, Mersmann S, Kersting M: Convenience foods in children's diet and association with dietary quality and body weight status. Eur J Clin Nutr 2011;65:160–166.
48 Looney SM, Raynor HA: Impact of portion size and energy density on snack intake in preschool-aged children. J AM DIET Assoc 2011;111:414–418.
49 McConahy KL, Smiciklas-Wright H, Mitchell DC, Picciano MF: Portion size of common foods predicts energy intake among preschool-aged children. J AM DIET Assoc 2004;104:975–979.
50 Monteiro CA: Nutrition and health. The issue is not food, nor nutrients, so much as processing. Publ Health Nutr 2009;12:729–731.
51 Keith SW, Redden DT, Katzmarzyk PT, Boggiano MM, Hanlon EC, et al: Putative contributors to the secular increase in obesity: exploring the roads less traveled. Int J Obes (Lond) 2006;30:1585–1594.
52 Westenhöfer J: Energy density and cost of foods in Germany. Ernährungs Umschau International 2013; 60:30–35.
53 Osei-Assibey G, Dick S, Macdiarmid J, Semple S, Reilly JJ, et al: The influence of the food environment on overweight and obesity in young children: a systematic review. BMJ Open 2012;2:e001538.
54 Muckelbauer R, Libuda L, Clausen K, Toschke AM, Reinehr T, et al: Promotion and provision of drinking water in schools for overweight prevention: randomized, controlled cluster trial. Pediatrics 2009; 123:e661–e667.
55 Savage JS, Mitchell DC, Smiciklas-Wright H, Symons Downs D, Birch LL: Plausible reports of energy intake may predict body mass index in pre-adolescent girls. J AM DIET Assoc 2008;108:131–135.
56 Prentice AM, Jebb SA: Fast foods, energy density and obesity: a possible mechanistic link. Obes Rev 2003; 4:187–194.
57 U.S. Department of Agriculture and U.S. Department of Health and Human Services Dietary Guidelines for Americans, 2010, ed 7. Washington, DC: U.S. Government Printing Office Publishing House.
58 Pérez-Escamilla R, Obbagy JE, Altman JM, Essery EV, McGrane MM, et al: Dietary energy density and body weight in adults and children: a systematic review. J Acad Nutr Diet 2012;112:671–684.
59 Bechthold A: Food energy density and body weight. Ernährungs Umschau International 2014;61:2–11.
60 Kranz S, Brauchla M, Slavin JL, Miller KB: What do we know about dietary fiber intake in children and health? The effects of fiber intake on constipation, obesity, and diabetes in children. Adv Nutr 2012;3: 47–53.

61 Muckelbauer R, Sarganas G, Grüneis A, Müller-Nordhorn J: Association between water consumption and body weight outcomes: a systematic review. Am J Clin Nutr 2013;98:282–289.
62 Diethelm K, Günther AL, Schulze MB, Standl M, Heinrich J, et al: Prospective relevance of dietary patterns at the beginning and during the course of primary school to the development of body composition. Br J Nutr 2014;2:1488–1498.
63 Hilbig A, Lentze MJ, Kersting M: Introduction and composition of complementary feeding. Scientific evidence and practical guidelines in Germany. Monatsschr Kinderheilkd 2012;160:1089–1095.
64 Mesch CM, Stimming M, Foterek K, Hilbig A, Alexy U, et al: Food variety in commercial and homemade complementary meals for infants in Germany. Market survey and dietary practice. Appetite 2014;76: 113–119.
65 ESPGHAN Committee on Nutrition, Agostoni C, Braegger C, Decsi T, Kolacek S, et al: Role of dietary factors and food habits in the development of childhood obesity: a commentary by the ESPGHAN Committee on Nutrition. J Pediatr Gastroenterol Nutr 2011;52:662–669.
66 Kersting M, Alexy U, Clausen K: Using the concept of food based dietary guidelines to develop an optimized mixed diet (OMD) for German children and adolescents. J Pediatr Gastroenterol Nutr 2005;40: 301–309.
67 EFSA NDA Panel: Scientific opinion on nutrient requirements and dietary intakes of infants and young children in the European Union. EFSA Journal 2013; 11:10.
68 Müller K, Clausen K, Pellmaier J, Krämer C, Kalhoff H, et al: Development and implementation of a children's menu according to the criteria of the optimised mixed diet in a paediatric hospital – a feasibility study. Ernährungs Umschau International 2013; 60:216–221.
69 Van Stralen MM, te Velde SJ, van Nassau F, Brug J, Grammatikaki E, et al: Weight status of European preschool children and associations with family demographics and energy balance-related behaviours: a pooled analysis of six European studies. Obes Rev 2012;13(Suppl):29–41.

Hermann Kalhoff, MD, PhD
Westfälisches Kinderzentrum
Beurhausstrasse 40
DE–44137 Bonn (Germany)
E-Mail hermann.kalhoff@klinikumdo.de

Kiess W, Wabitsch M, Maffeis C, Sharma AM (eds): Metabolic Syndrome and Obesity in Childhood and Adolescence.
Pediatr Adolesc Med. Basel, Karger, 2015, vol 19, pp 53–67 (DOI: 10.1159/000368124)

Sedentary Lifestyle

Augustin Raupp • Béatrice Jouret • Maïthé Tauber

Hôpital des Enfants and the Network for Prevention and Care of Paediatric Obesity, CHU Toulouse, Toulouse, France

Abstract

According to the World Health Organisation, sedentary behaviour is the fourth highest risk factor for mortality in the world today, with many aspects of our society contributing to increasingly sedentary lifestyles. Sedentary behaviour (low energy expenditure, or ≤1.5 metabolic equivalents of task in a situation of arousal) should be distinguished from inactivity, which is characterised by failure to reach the recommended physical activity levels. The most pernicious sedentary behaviour is the time spent in front of screens. Regardless of the level of physical activity, screen time is associated with decreases in physical fitness, self-esteem, and academic performance and an increase in cardiovascular and metabolic risk. Several publications have shown that 80.3% of 13–15 year olds are physically active for less than 60 min per day and that 67% spend at least 2 h per day watching television. Prevention strategies should focus on environmental determinants (physical and social), particularly in the family model. Some of the current research focuses on the use of new technologies (augmented reality) as an educational tool.

Introduction and Definitions

Context

Perhaps nothing is as natural to us as physical activity. With no exaggeration, one might even say that we have been 'programmed' to move. It should therefore be surprising to no one to learn that physical activity contributes not only to children's psychomotor development but also to their deepest sense of well-being. Infancy is a critical time of life for building the behavioural patterns that will result in an active or sedentary lifestyle [1], but the problem of sedentary behaviour is quite complex.

From prehistoric times to the 1850s, humans were physically active essentially by necessity: to eat and build shelter. From then on, it became increasingly possible to meet such basic needs with far less physical effort. The notion of leisure began to spread, and physical activity became diversified to include relaxation and pleasure and even competition and performance as the sports movement gradually took hold.

In today's world, the quality of life is declining in certain populations, and for many, meeting basic needs is a major preoccupation. For the most vulnerable among us, dealing with 'day-to-day emergencies' has become increasingly complicated and the sources of pleasure increasingly hard to find.

Deconditioning is often understood in terms of physical activity, but it may begin as a psychological phenomenon, such as when the ongoing stress of daily living alters an individual's capacity to cope and make wise choices and generally undermines the ability to call upon personal resources. When this point has been reached, it becomes difficult to see making an (physical) effort as a means to pleasure. Pleasure has been considered in terms of the norms of the world in which we live, and in this case, even pleasure should be 'consumable' on demand.

Marketing strategies have indeed been built around this notion, which is amply displayed by the marketing of video games, reality shows, and other types of passive leisure activities based on video screens and virtual worlds. Well-being no longer derives from physically moving, and creative capacities have become inhibited. For sedentary youth, screen time has become a way to feel competent and build a sense of self-worth, and therefore, we need to acknowledge it as a relatively new source of pleasure and personal satisfaction [2].

Physical activity, in contrast, has become a kind of discipline; it is perceived as a type of leisure activity for when there is enough time. Most of us know that it is a route to good health, but it takes energy and discipline to fit it into daily life.

Society today is therefore showing a tendency to 'deprogram' the innate need to move by offering in its place a multitude of attractive alternatives that encourage sedentary behaviour in younger and younger children. It actually may seem easier today to adopt a sedentary lifestyle instead of an active one, even for the very youngest among us. Socialisation processes have changed with our increasing dependence on technology: as the internet has become accessible to almost all, the way that we socialise has become increasingly virtual, especially for adolescents.

With the internet, geographical boundaries no longer limit the creation and maintenance of social relationships: nearly the whole world is available for direct interaction. The great paradox in all of this is that in order to move faster, we no longer move at all. Youth especially often feel as if they are actors in a virtual reality, in which some of them truly become lost.

In this chapter, we first define the terms that we will be using. We then look at some of the statistics on sedentary behaviour in young people as well as the health consequences and, especially, the risk factors for cardiometabolic disease and obesity. We attempt to determine which factors influence the adoption of sedentary behaviours and which types of interventions are most effective in countering these behaviours in youth.

Definitions and Evaluation

Sedentary behaviour has been recognised as a public health issue for only the past 10 years [3]. However, according to the World Health Organisation, it is the fourth biggest risk factor for mortality in the world. One of the greatest difficulties for public health officials is the lack of consensus in the literature about what sedentary behaviour is as opposed to inactivity and how to define the various types of sedentary behaviour.

Sedentary behaviour is often defined as low energy expenditure (≤1.5 metabolic equivalents of task) and a sitting or reclining posture. However, the literature on sports and physical exercise generally defines this behaviour as failure to meet the recommended thresholds for physical activity (60 min of moderate to vigorous physical activity (MVPA) per day for children). It may therefore be worthwhile to distinguish low energy expenditure due to excessive sitting and reclining from not meeting the physical activity guidelines.

Tremblay and the Sedentary Behaviours Research Network have therefore proposed standardised definitions of 'sedentary', 'sedentary behaviour', and 'inactive' [4].

Sedentary behaviour is characterised by low energy expenditure (≤1.5 metabolic equivalents of task) and a seated or lying-down position during waking hours.

A person is sedentary when his or her behaviour is mostly sedentary and the person exceeds the recommended maximum time in front of a television (TV) or computer screen (2 h for 5–17 year olds, as suggested in a literature review by Tremblay et al. [5]).

'Inactive' defines those individuals who perform insufficient amounts of MVPA and are thus not meeting the guidelines.

It should therefore be kept in mind that prolonged sitting and not meeting the recommendations for MVPA are independent risk factors. In addition, reducing the amount of sedentary time does not automatically mean an increase in the quantity of physical activity. The two factors therefore need to be carefully evaluated in tandem on a regular basis.

We will see further on that it is also important to distinguish screen time, and particularly watching TV, from other sedentary behaviours because screen time has an independent impact compared with other risk factors. Most often, screen time is evaluated by questionnaire and is thus a self-report measure.

Daily energy expenditure and periods of being completely sedentary (not just screen time) are currently assessed by accelerometry, which is not a robust method, as it does not take posture into account. Sitting and standing at rest are physiologically different because they do not require the same energy expenditure. There are considerable disparities in the threshold values used to determine and evaluate sedentary behaviour by the use of accelerometers (from 100 to 1,100 cycles per minute, depending on the study) [6].

Epidemiology: Some Striking Figures

A major review of the literature [7] presented data from 105 countries that had participated in two international studies on adolescent physical activity: the Global School-based Student Health Survey [8] and the Health Behaviour in School-aged Children study [9]. The main findings were as follows:

- In total, 80.3% of 13–15 year olds were physically active for less than 60 min per day and could thus be described as inactive.
- Additionally, 66% of the boys and 68% of the girls from among the 13–15 year olds spent at least 2 h per day watching TV and thus had excessively sedentary behaviour.

Physical activity and sedentary behaviour have been extensively studied as health determinants in Canada. Some of the studies have included a broad range of ages and have shown that only 7% of children, adolescents, and young adults from 6 to 19 years old perform at least 60 min of MVPA per day. Canadian children spend an average of 8.6 h per day being sedentary, which amounts to 62% of their waking hours [10]. It is important to examine the types of sedentary behaviour, however, as their impacts on health may differ.

Another Canadian study showed that children with an average age of 10.7 years spent an average of 3.3 h per day (3.1 h during the week and 3.6 h on the weekend) on screen-related activities, with 74% exceeding the recommended limit of 2 h per day. Boys spent more time on these activities because they played more video games [11].

The American National Health and Nutrition Examination Survey indicated that nearly half (47%) of children aged between 2 and 15 years exceeded this recommendation [12]. A difference related to weight status was noted: 58.5% of obese youth, as opposed to 44.6% of normal-weight youth, spent more than 2 h in front of screens.

A Spanish study of 3,503 adolescents from 12 to 18 years old reported that 46% of the girls and 26% of the boys did not meet the physical activity recommendations [13].

The considerable differences in the figures according to the study and the country strongly suggest the need to standardise the evaluation instruments and thresholds for objective measures.

The Spanish study reported an interesting finding that suggests a link between sedentary behaviour and the physical activity level: the boys who reported a total screen time of ≥4 h per day had a 64% greater risk of not meeting the minimum for physical activity. The total screen time was negatively associated with the physical activity level among the boys. Participation in supervised activities, however, seemed to counteract the negative impact of screen time. Children and adolescents who participated in structured activities were overall more physically active than those who participated in spontaneous and self-organised activities.

The Link between Sedentary Behaviour and Obesity, Risk Factors, and Other Health Problems

It has been well established that regardless of the physical activity level, sedentary behaviours are associated with an increased risk of all-cause mortality, cardiometabolic disease, and many other physiological and psychological problems [14–16].

In a review of the literature, Tremblay et al. [5] found a dose-response relationship between an increase in sedentary behaviour and an unfavourable health status in young people. The sedentary behaviour with the most negative impact on health was TV viewing. In total, 94 studies showed that an increase in sedentary behaviour had an impact on at least one of the following health indicators: fat mass, body mass index (BMI), and risk of overweight.

For example, a study of 461 Mexican children showed that the risk of obesity rose by 12% for each hour of TV viewing reported on a self-response questionnaire [17]. Another longitudinal study [18] of children and adolescents aged between 9 and 15 years and in the 50th, 75th, or 90th percentile on the weight curve demonstrated that objectively measured sedentary time was a risk factor for weight gain, independent of other factors, like food intake, the physical activity level, and sleep. In another study of adolescents, every additional hour of TV viewing was associated with a 0.22 kg/m^2 increase in BMI [19]. In addition, the prevalence of back pain increased by 10% for every extra hour in front of a computer, TV, or video game [20].

The HELENA study [21] revealed that boys who spent more than 4 h per day playing video games on the weekend had a higher risk of metabolic disease, independent of obesity.

With regard to the dose-response relationship, spending more than 2 h per day watching TV was also correlated with the following:

- A decline in physical fitness, and specifically aerobic aptitude (a drop in VO_2 max) and cardiorespiratory and musculoskeletal aptitudes.
- An increase in the risk of cardiovascular disease and metabolic syndrome (high cholesterol, arterial blood pressure, HbA1c, and insulin resistance).
- A drop in self-esteem and prosocial behaviour. Another review of the adolescent literature reported that 75% of studies showed a decrease in socialising time in association with increased sedentary time [22].
- Lower school performance and capacity for attention/concentration, with some particularly disturbing correlations:
  - between 1 and 2 h of TV viewing per day: difficulty in paying attention
  - more than 2 h per day: a drop in school grades
  - more than 3 h per day: a drop in school performance and low IQ

With regard to psychological indicators, three studies reported a positive association between sedentary time and depressive syndrome [23–25]. In addition, four studies reported a negative association with perceived health status: as the sedentary time increased, the perceived health status and psychosocial well-being declined [25–28].

Mechanisms Explaining How Screen Time Increases Adiposity

Two mechanisms may explain how screen time increases adiposity: screen time reduces the time spent on physical activity [29] and increases energy intake [30–32]. The second association has been the focus of several recent studies. Spending time watching TV has been associated with the consumption of foods with high calorie density, and this association seems to be increased by TV advertising [33–35]. When children watch televised food advertisements, they increase food intake by 45% when they are allowed to eat freely [36]. This effect is particularly striking in overweight and obese youth, who have shown a better capacity than normal-weight youth to remember advertising messages [37].

Even without food advertising, food intake increases to the same degree [38, 39]. With new technologies like smartphones and tablets, young people have access to video content without advertising and thus have greater control over what they watch [40]. Moreover, they often watch more than one screen at a time (46% of them do something else while watching TV), particularly during commercial breaks [41]. Adolescents thus take advantage of having several choices, and they filter out unwanted content like commercials [42].

Mekhmoukh et al. showed that watching TV while eating increased food intake by 10%, but only in overweight adolescents [43]. In normal-weight adolescents, Peneau et al. [44] found that food intake did not increase, although soda intake increased significantly.

Some studies have specifically investigated the mechanisms by which energy intake is increased:

- Bellissimo et al. [45] found that watching TV while eating alters the physiological signals of satiety and satiation. In boys, glucose absorption before a meal did not diminish the quantity of food intake when eating while watching TV.
- In girls, Patel [46] showed that the impact of environmental factors on food intake depends on pubertal status: quantities remained unchanged in postpubertal girls while watching TV but increased in peripubertal girls.

Chaput [47] also showed that food intake increased by 80 kcal during meals among adolescent boys after they had played passive video games compared with those who had been sitting but doing nothing. This might be explained by the stimulation of the stress-induced reward system caused by playing video games. Further research is needed to investigate this hypothesis.

Determinants of Sedentary Behaviour

Age

Sedentary behaviour tends to increase with age. In Canada, children under 11 years of age spend about 1.3 h less on sedentary behaviours than adolescents between 11 and 14 years old do and 2 h less than adolescents from 15 to 19 years old do [10].

Early adolescence is therefore a critical period because it is associated with an increase in physical inactivity [48, 49]. Longitudinal studies have shown that screen time as well as the total sedentary time especially increase during this period. A British survey notably revealed that in the 5 years after entering adolescence, the weekly time spent in front of screens increased by 2.5 h. This was matched by a significant decrease in physical activity that was more marked in girls (46% less, as opposed to 23% for boys) [48]. Moreover, habits that develop at this age tend to persist into adulthood [50].

Gender

Girls watch more TV than boys do, and their physical activity level declines more noticeably in adolescence. Girls are also more prone to depression, anxiety, and low self-esteem. These variables can favour or aggravate high levels of sedentary behaviour [51, 52].

The HELENA study [21] confirmed these results, showing that boys engage in more sustained physical activity than girls do. Boys also show a greater tendency to enrol in supervised activities. However, they watch more TV in their bedrooms and play more video games.

Socioeconomic Status

Before the age of 7 years, socioeconomic status is consistently found to be associated with screen time. Low status is associated with high screen time and, especially, TV viewing [53]. Other leisure-time activities are usually offered in homes with higher socioeconomic status.

Another study [54] of 3,822 English children aged from 5 to 15 years showed that when the focus was on overall sedentary behaviour, children from a high socioeconomic position were in fact more sedentary but were sedentary while engaged in leisure activities other than TV viewing. TV is therefore not an indicator for reliable estimations of the total sedentary time, but the type of sedentary behaviour counts more than the total sedentary time since we have seen that it is particularly harmful to spend time watching TV.

One study showed that a low maternal educational level was associated with children viewing more than 2 h of TV per day. This same study also showed associations between maternal BMI and TV viewing time as well as between maternal smoking and viewing time [55].

Many studies have shown discrepant results concerning the association between the total TV viewing time and whether mothers work. The assumption is that stay-at-home mothers are better able to supervise their children's TV viewing time, but this has not been systematically shown to be the case.

The study cited above [55] emphasised the crucial role of parents even in infancy, as more and more children are walked in a stroller instead of walking themselves.

Parental Habits and Family Impact

In young children from 3 to 5 years old, one study [56] showed that environmental factors contributed to the development of sedentary behaviours. As in other developmental areas, the parental lifestyle encourages certain behaviours in children. Some authors have specifically investigated parents' sedentary behaviours, their capacity to set limits on their children's screen time, and the amount of multimedia equipment in the home. The findings were as follows: two thirds of the children and three quarters of the parents spent 2 or more hours watching TV per day. The children whose parents spent more than 2 h watching TV were five times more likely to also spend more than 2 h in front of the TV. The parents reported low perceived self-efficacy for physical activity, but they also reported that they were capable of encouraging physical activity in their children and limiting their children's screen time. This finding suggests that many parents do not grasp the influence that their own behaviour has on their children or that because they themselves are sedentary, they are unaware of the recommendations. Perceived self-efficacy had a powerful impact on the children's TV viewing time because each additional point on the evaluation scale was associated with a 77% drop in the probability that the child would spend more than 2 h watching TV.

Half of the families reported owning more than 11 multimedia devices. As the number of devices in the home rose, so did the time that the parents spent watching TV.

A study conducted in Ontario primary schools [11] found that most of the children watched TV and played video games for entertainment but that more than half of them also reported playing video games out of boredom. The children with more than 2 h of screen time per day highlight a new mode of socialising through the use of these media. Half of the children reported that their parents set limits on screen time during the week, but barely one third had limits set on the weekend. Fully 80% of the parents stated that it was important to control the amount of time that their children watch TV, and 64% indicated that they do not allow their children to make these daily decisions.

Environmental Determinants

Rural/Urban

To investigate the environmental factors affecting sedentary behaviour, an Australian study focused specifically on mothers [57]. Those living in rural areas reported better access to physical activity equipment in the home, better physical activity performances from their children, better relations with neighbours, better social networks, and better perceived safety in the proximal environment.

Bruner [58] studied 5,000 Canadian adolescents and showed that the place of residence made no difference to the amount of physical activity, but this study did find that young children in rural areas had less screen time that those in big cities after adjustment for socioeconomic status. The social networks in cities were found to favour sedentary behaviour, whereas these networks showed a tendency to reduce this behaviour in rural areas. The children in rural areas played outdoors more often.

A study of 3,000 American children [59] revealed that the children living in small towns had the highest physical activity levels, followed by children in rural areas. The Rural-Urban Continuum Codes [60] were used to assess the population densities.

Timperio [61] showed that screen time rose with an increase in traffic density. Safe roads are reassuring to parents, who are then more apt to let their children go out more often. This in turn may increase physical activity if children walk to their destinations.

An English study [62] showed that because of increased concerns about safety in urban areas, longer parental working hours, and greater distances to travel, only 9% of children were allowed to walk to school unaccompanied in 1991 as opposed to 80% in 1971. These figures, which date back more than 20 years, suggest the powerful impact of the physical environment on the sedentary behaviour of youth. Similar results have been reported in other European countries.

The Physical Environment in the Home and the Relationship between Physical and Social Environments

Concerning the physical environment in the home, a literature review entitled 'A place for play' [63] showed that the amount of multimedia equipment is positively correlated with sedentary behaviour in young people. Nine observational studies out of 18 showed the same relationship when multimedia equipment was in the bedroom. However, the associations were not objectively measured by accelerometry.

This review also studied the relationships between environmental, social, and physical factors in the home. A certain number of elements were confirmed: in particular, certain types of family social support were positively associated with sedentary behaviour. For example, parental use of multimedia electronics was correlated with children's use.

Management and Prevention

Parental habits and the parental ability to set limits on children's screen time seem to affect the sedentary behaviours of their children. The above review [63] analysed different types of interventions and showed that making and enforcing rules was effective because having rules was directly correlated with a lower level of sedentary behaviour (11 studies out of 14). These studies of interventions to limit TV viewing time showed good results, with an improvement in BMI in two of the studies and an increase in physical activity in one of them. For example, a study by Robinson [62] showed that an intervention to reduce screen time in elementary school children resulted in a 2.3 cm decrease in waist circumference and a 0.45 kg/m^2 drop in BMI after 6 months.

Changing the physical environment can influence the level of physical activity and sedentary behaviours. It has not, however, been demonstrated that reducing the amount of multimedia equipment in the home helps children to be less sedentary because they tend to simply replace one sedentary behaviour with another.

The most convincing intervention results were found in the social environment, with parents having the most crucial role, even when the physical environment was not in itself conducive to greater physical activity.

Another type of intervention makes use of active video games, which have become quite sophisticated, although most randomised controlled trials have shown that their use has no effect on the total time spent on physical activity [64]. Indeed, no significant difference was found in the physical activity level after 12 weeks for those who received an intervention of active video gaming compared with those who played passive video games. A few rare studies have shown a short-term increase in physical activity, but this then decreases. Active video games therefore are not an effective solution for combating obesity. They do not measurably contribute to the 60 min of daily MVPA recommended for children.

In addition, these games are quite attractive to children in the beginning, but interest tends to fade quickly. Intrinsic motivation continues to be stronger for conventional fitness courses. The one valuable aspect of these games is that they help children to acquire certain motor skills.

Only one video game (Dance Dance Revolution) seemed to show satisfactory results, with studies reporting an increase in overall weekly energy expenditure and VO_2 max. The effect on adiposity and weight gain was moderate, with a greater effect on overweight or obese people. In contrast, no significant result has been found for cardiometabolic indicators, including triglyceride levels, high-density lipoprotein and low-density lipoprotein cholesterol, insulin sensitivity, and glucose tolerance. Energy intakes were also not affected.

The types of interventions that have shown the most interesting results were those in which obtaining time to watch TV or play video games was determined by the amount of prior physical activity. However, the long-term effects of these interventions have not been assessed, and this approach does not seem consistent with the principles of prevention and obesity management. Indeed, one of the main goals is to help young people to build a strong association between physical activity and pleasure. In contrast, making the amount of physical activity a condition for obtaining screen time introduces a constraint (having to be physically active) that must be endured in order to obtain pleasure (watching TV). In this scenario, moving is not pleasure in itself but is performed only to obtain a reward.

Public health researchers are developing new intervention strategies using screen-based technologies that can become part of the solution rather than the problem. Manipulating the game environment as a tool for interventions targeting increased

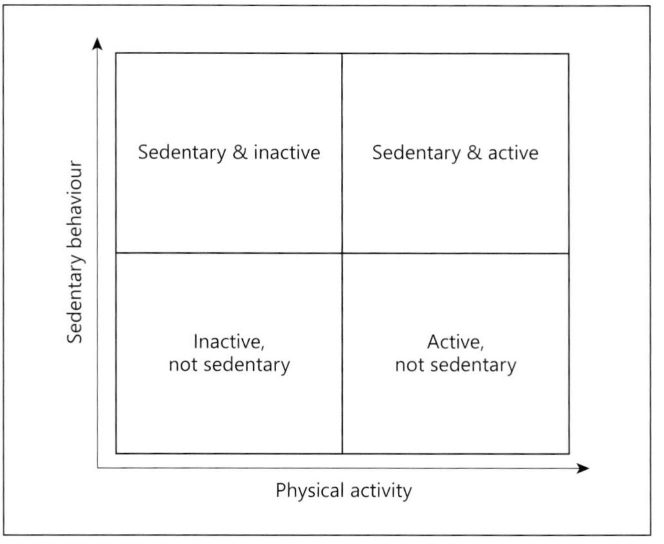

Fig. 1. Sedentary behaviour and physical activity as distinct constructs. With permission form Saunders et al. [64].

physical activity is one such example. In this type of intervention, based on new-generation applications of 'augmented reality', users act through the superposition of virtual information on their own perceptions of reality.

Most randomised controlled trials have shown little change in the usual physical activity level, however. These new tools nevertheless continue to be developed and are in constant evolution. Further evaluation will undoubtedly be needed in the future.

Discussion and Conclusion

Sedentary behaviours have dramatically increased in youth over the last 20 years. The research on the health effects of the sedentary lifestyle has clearly demonstrated that sedentary behaviour is an independent risk factor for cardiometabolic disease. Moreover, it is now well documented that activity/inactivity and sedentary behaviour are two distinct variables (see fig. 1 below) [64].

We now know that sedentary behaviour is directly linked to the markers of adiposity. The reported screen time, rather than the objectively measured total sedentary time, is associated with cardiometabolic disease risk [65].

Further and more extensive research is needed, especially into the characteristics of sedentary behaviours in children, the threshold definitions for objective accelerometric measurement, and the most effective interventions to limit sedentary behaviours.

The influence of the family is primordial and thus is the priority for focus. Sedentary behaviour is more prevalent in families with low socioeconomic status. Most of the children who watch TV for an average of more than 2 h per day perceive a lack of parental control over weekend screen time [11].

Generally, we note good awareness of the harmful effects of sedentary lifestyles and the importance of physical activity. This highlights the difference between attitude and behaviour. The mode of evaluation (questionnaire) usually deals with explicit, and not implicit, attitudes. Children under ecological conditions are, however, more attentive to their 'implicit needs', and they do not perform a cost-benefit analysis.

Many parents explain that their children are under pressure from peers and advertising and that they then put this pressure on their parents. These parents find it difficult to take a stand and thus have a hard time setting limits. The parents of preschool children say that they are more concerned with what their children watch than with how much time they spend watching. When their children are this young, parents also seem less aware of the risk of obesity linked to screen time. Additionally, some parents think that their children get enough physical activity from active video games because they see them moving, and in a reassuring context: the home.

In the last decade, some authors have hypothesised that adiposity determines the physical activity level and not the converse, as has long been assumed. Longitudinal studies [66, 67] have indeed shown that the physical activity level at the start of the studies did not predict changes in adiposity, although the basal adiposity was a factor contributing to sedentary time.

Last, just as physical activity needs to be promoted in a variety of ways, changes in management and prevention strategies must occur at several levels. It is first essential that interventions target parents to strengthen perceived self-efficacy and enhance their awareness of just how great an impact their own behaviour has on their children. It is also important to act in terms of the physical and geographic environment to address parental feelings of insecurity, to provide greater access to adapted and supervised playgrounds, and therefore to encourage parents to push outdoor activities. Moreover, although it is important to avoid taking a moralising tone or stigmatising sedentary behaviour as somehow 'deviant', we need to encourage and assist our young in learning to find pleasure in what may be, for them, a 'new' way: by being truly active in the world. However, this will have to be done while taking into account the actual lifestyles of youth today and the technological developments in virtual reality and augmented reality. These new tools may in fact be harnessed one day to encourage the capacity to truly become an actor in one's own life and to play an active role in one's health.

References

1 Janz KF, Burns TL, Levy SM: Tracking of activity and sedentary behaviors in childhood. The Iowa Bone Development Study. Am J Prev Med 2005;29:171–178.

2 Puglisi LM, Okely AD, Pearson P, et al: Barriers to increasing physical activity and limiting small screen recreation among obese children. Obes Res Clin Pract 2010;4:e33–e40.

3 Levine JA, Lanningham-Foster LM, McCrady SK, et al: Interindividual variation in posture allocation: possible role in human obesity. Science 2005;307:584–586.

4 Sedentary Behaviour Research Network: Letter to the editor: standardized use of the terms 'sedentary' and 'sedentary behaviours'. Appl Physiol Nutr Metab Physiol 2012;37:540–542.

5 Tremblay MS, LeBlanc AG, Kho ME, et al: Systematic review of sedentary behaviour and health indicators in school-aged children and youth. Int J Behav Nutr Phys Act 2011;8:98–120.
6 Atkin AJ, Ekelund U, Møller NC, et al: Sedentary time in children: influence of accelerometer processing on health relations. Med Sci Sports Exerc 2012; 45:1097–1104.
7 Hallal PC, Andersen LB, Bull FC, et al: Global physical activity levels: surveillance progress, pitfalls, and prospects. Lancet 2012;380:247–257.
8 WHO: Global school-based student health survey. 2011. http://www.who.int/chp/gshs/en/ (accessed March 23, 2012).
9 WHO Regional Office for Europe: Inequalities in young people's health: HBSC international report from the 2005/2006 survey. Copenhagen, WHO Regional Office for Europe, 2008.
10 Colley RC, Garriguet D, Janssen I, et al: Physical activity of Canadian children and youth: accelerometer results from the 2007 to 2009 Canadian Health Measures Survey. Health Rep 2011;22:15–24.
11 He M, Piche L, Beynon C, et al: Screen-related sedentary behaviors: children's and parents' attitudes, motivations, and practices. J Nutr Educ Behav 2010; 42:17–25.
12 Sisson SB, Church TS, Martin CK, et al: Profiles of sedentary behavior in children and adolescents: the US National Health and Nutrition Examination Survey, 2001–2006. Int J Pediatr Obes 2009;4:353–359.
13 Serrano-Sanchez JA, Martí-Trujillo S, Lera-Navarro A, et al: Associations between screen time and physical activity among Spanish adolescents. PLoS ONE 2011;6:e24453.
14 Treuth MS, Catellier DJ, Schmitz KH, et al: Weekend and weekday patterns of physical activity in overweight and normal-weight adolescent girls. Obesity (Silver Spring) 2007;15:1782–1788.
15 Katzmarzyk PT, Church TS, Craig CL, et al: Sitting time and mortality from all causes, cardiovascular disease, and cancer. Med Sci Sports Exerc 2009;41: 998–1005.
16 Owen N, Bauman A, Brown W: Too much sitting: a novel and important predictor of chronic disease risk? Br J Sports Med 2009;43:81–83.
17 Hernández B, Gortmaker SL, Colditz GA, et al: Association of obesity with physical activity, television programs and other forms of video viewing among children in Mexico city. Int J Obes Relat Metab Disord 1999;23:845–854.
18 Mitchell JA, Pate RR, Beets MW, et al: Time spent in sedentary behavior and changes in childhood BMI: a longitudinal study from ages 9 to 15 years. Int J Obes 2013;37:54–60.
19 Hu FB: Overweight and obesity in women: Health risks and consequences. J Womens Health 2003;12: 163–172.
20 Torsheim T, Eriksson L, Schnohr C, et al: Screen-based activities and physical complaints among adolescents from the Nordic countries. BMC Public Health 2010;10:324.
21 Rey-López JP, Bel-Serrat S, Santaliestra-Pasias A, et al: Sedentary behaviour and clustered metabolic risk in adolescents: The HELENA study. Nutr Metab Cardiovasc Dis 2012;23:1017–1024.
22 Costigan SA, Barnett L, Plotnikoff RC, et al: The health indicators associated with screen-based sedentary behavior among adolescent girls: a systematic review. J Adolesc Health 2013;52:382–392.
23 Hume C, Timperio A, Veitch J, et al: Physical activity, sedentary behavior, and depressive symptoms among adolescents. J Phys Activity Health 2011;8: 152–156.
24 Bélanger RE, Akre C, Berchtold A, et al: A U-shaped association between intensity of internet use and adolescent health. Pediatrics 2011;127:e330–e335.
25 Brodersen N, Steptoe A, Williamson S, et al: Sociodemographic, developmental, environmental, and psychological correlates of physical activity and sedentary behavior at age 11 to 12. Ann Behav Med 2005; 29:2–11.
26 Ussher M, Owen C, Cook D, et al: The relationship between physical activity, sedentary behaviour and psychological wellbeing among adolescents. Soc Psychiatry Psychiatric Epidemiol 2007;42:851–856.
27 Punamäki R-L, Wallenius M, Nygård C-H, et al: Use of information and communication technology (ICT) and perceived health in adolescence: the role of sleeping habits and waking-time tiredness. J Adolesc 2007;30:569–585.
28 Jackson LA, von Eye A, Fitzgerald HE, et al: Self-concept, self-esteem, gender, race and information technology use. Computers Human Behav 2010;26:323–328.
29 Jenvey V: The relationship between television viewing and obesity in young children. A review of existing explanations. Early Child Development and Care 2007;177:809–820.
30 Boulos R, Vikre EK, Oppenheimer S, et al: ObesiTV. How television is influencing the obesity epidemic. Physiol Behav 2012;107:146–153.
31 Hastings G, Stead M, McDermott L, et al: Review of Research on the Effects of Food Promotion to Children. Glasgow, Centre for Social Marketing, University of Strathclyde, 2003.
32 Robinson TN: Television viewing and childhood obesity. Pediatr Clin North Am 2001;48:1017–1025.
33 Effertz T, Wilcke A-C: Do television food commercials target children in Germany. Public Health Nutr 2012;15:1466–1473.

34 Haug E, Rasmussen M, Samdal O, et al: Overweight in school-aged children and its relationship with demographic and lifestyle factors. Results from the WHO-Collaborative Health Behaviour in School-aged Children (HBSC) study. Int J Public Health 2009;54(suppl 2):167–179.
35 Kelly B, Chapman K, King L, et al: Trends in food advertising to children on free-to-air television in Australia. Aust N Z J Public Health 2011;35:131–134.
36 Harris JL, Bargh JA, Brownell KD: Priming effects of television food advertising on eating behavior. Health Psychol 2009;28:404–413.
37 Halford JC, Gillespie J, Brown V, et al: Effect of television advertisements for foods on food consumption in children. Appetite 2004;42:221–225.
38 Chaput J-P, Klingenberg L, Astrup A, et al: Modern sedentary activities promote overconsumption of food in our current obesogenic environment. Obes Rev 2011;12:e12–e20.
39 Volkow ND, Wang GJ, Fowler JS, et al: Food and drug reward. Overlapping circuits in human obesity and addiction. Curr Top Behav Neurosci 2012;11:1–24.
40 Carlson M: Tapping into TiVo. Digital video recorders and the transition from schedules to surveillance in television. New Media Soc 2006;8:97–115.
41 Schmitt KL, Woolf KD, Anderson DR: Viewing the viewers. Viewing behaviors by children and adults during television programs and commercials. J Commun 2003;53:265–281.
42 Jago R, Sebire SJ, Gorely T, et al: I'm on it 24/7 at the moment. A qualitative examination of multi-screen viewing behaviours among UK 10–11 year olds. Int J Behav Nutr Phys Act 2011;8:85.
43 Mekhmoukh A, Chapelot D, Bellisle F: Influence of environmental factors on meal intake in overweight and normal-weight male adolescents. A laboratory study. Appetite 2012;59:90–95.
44 Peneau S, Mekhmoukh A, Chapelot D, et al: Influence of environmental factors on food intake and choice of beverage during meals in teenagers. A laboratory study. Br J Nutr 2009;102:1854–1859.
45 Bellissimo N, Pencharz PB, Thomas SG, et al: Effect of television viewing at mealtime on food intake after a glucose preload in boys. Pediatr Res 2007;61:745–749.
46 Patel BP, Bellissimo N, Thomas SG, et al: Television viewing at mealtime reduces caloric compensation in peripubertal, but not postpubertal, girls. Pediatr Res 2011;70:513–517.
47 Chaput JP, Visby T, Nyby S, et al: Video game playing increases food intake in adolescents: a randomized crossover study. Am J Clin Nutr 2011;93:1196–1203.
48 Brodersen NH, Steptoe A, Boniface DR, et al: Trends in physical activity and sedentary behaviour in adolescence: ethnic and socioeconomic differences. Br J Sports Med 2007;41:140–144.
49 Elder JP, Lytle L, Sallis JF, et al: A description of the social-ecological framework used in the Trial of Activity for Adolescent Girls (TAAG). Health Educ Res 2007;22:155–165.
50 Hardy LL, Bass SL, Booth ML: Changes in sedentary behavior among adolescent girls: A 2.5-year prospective cohort study. J Adolesc Health 2007;40:158–165.
51 Boyd CP, Gullone E, Kostanski M, et al: Prevalence of anxiety and depression in Australian adolescents: comparisons with worldwide data. J Genet Psychol 2000;161:479–492.
52 Nihill GFJ, Lubans DR, Plotnikoff RC: Associations between sedentary behavior and self-esteem in adolescent girls from schools in low-income communities. Mental Health Phys Activity 2013;6:30–35.
53 van Rossem L, Vogel I, Moll HA, et al: An observational study on socio-economic and ethnic differences in indicators of sedentary behavior and physical activity in preschool children. Prev Med 2012;54:55–60.
54 Coombs N, Shelton N, Rowlands A, et al: Children's and adolescents' sedentary behavior in relation to socioeconomic position. J Epidemiol Community Health 2013;67:868–874.
55 Miller SA, Taveras EM, Rifas-Shiman SL, et al: Association between television viewing and poor diet quality in young children. Int J Pediatr Obes 2008;3:168–176.
56 Jago R, Sebire SJ, Edwards MJ, et al: Parental TV viewing, parental self-efficacy, media equipment and TV viewing among preschool children. Eur J Pediatr 2013;172:1543–1545.
57 Salmon J, Veitch J, Abbott G, et al: Are associations between the perceived home and neighbourhood environment and children's physical activity and sedentary behaviour moderated by urban/rural location? Health Place 2013;24:44–53.
58 Bruner MW, Lawson J, Pickett W, et al: Rural Canadian adolescents are more likely to be obese compared with urban adolescents. Int J Pediatr Obes 2008;3:205–211.
59 Joens-Matre RR, Welk GJ, Calabro MA, et al: Rural-urban differences in physical activity, physical fitness, and over-weight prevalence of children. J Rural Health 2008;24:49–54.
60 U.S. Dept. of Agriculture, Economic Research Service: Measuring rurality: rural-urban continuum Codes. 2005. http://www.ers.usda.gov/briefing/rurality/RuralUrbCon/ (accessed August 2, 2005).

61 Timperio A, Salmon J, Ball K, et al: Neighborhood characteristics and TV viewing in youth: nothing to do but watch TV? J Sci Med Sport 2012;15:122–128.
62 Hillman M, Adams J, Whitelegg J: Conclusions Chapter 6; in Hillman M, Adams J, Whitelegg J (eds): One False Move. A Study of Children's Independent Mobility. London, Policy Studies Institute, 1990.
63 Maitland C, Stratton G, Foster S, et al: A place for play? The influence of the home physical environment on children's physical activity and sedentary behaviour. Int J Behav Nutr Phys Act 2013;10:99.
64 Saunders TJ, Chaput JP, Tremblay MS: Sedentary behaviour as an emerging risk factor for cardiometabolic diseases in children and youth. Can J Diabetes 2014;38:53–61.
65 Carson V, Janssen I: Volume, patterns, and types of sedentary behavior and cardio-metabolic health in children and adolescents: a cross-sectional study. BMC Pub Health 2011;11:274.
66 Ekelund U, Brage S, Besson H, et al: Time spent being sedentary and weight gain in healthy adults: reverse or bidirectional causality? Am J Clin Nutr 2008;88:612–617.
67 Metcalf BS, Hosking J, Jeffery AN, et al: Fatness leads to inactivity, but inactivity does not lead to fatness: a longitudinal study in children. Arch Dis Child 2011; 96:942–947.

Augustin Raupp
RéPPOP Midi-Pyrénées, Hôpital des enfants – Unité d'endocrinologie
330, avenue de Grande Bretagne, TSA 70034
FR–31059 Toulouse Cedex 9 (France)
E-Mail raupp.a@chu-toulouse.fr

Kiess W, Wabitsch M, Maffeis C, Sharma AM (eds): Metabolic Syndrome and Obesity in Childhood and Adolescence.
Pediatr Adolesc Med. Basel, Karger, 2015, vol 19, pp 68–74 (DOI: 10.1159/000368106)

Socio-Economic Aspects

Sandra Plachta-Danielzik · Manfred James Müller
Institut für Humanernährung und Lebensmittelkunde, Christian-Albrechts-Universität zu Kiel, Kiel, Germany

Abstract
During the last 30 years, the prevalence of overweight has risen substantially. Within societies, the prevalence of overweight is not equally distributed among people. There are socio-economic differentials in lifestyle, overweight, and health: the lower the socio-economic status is, the more frequent unhealthy lifestyles and overweight and its co-morbidities are. The problem is not confined to the poorest people, but rather, the gradient is across the whole society. Socio-economic inequalities in overweight and health result from an unequal distribution of opportunities and resources within a society.

Introduction

In Western societies, considerable changes in lifestyles and living conditions have been observed during the last 30 years, affecting human health as well as our environment. There has been a considerable increase in the prevalence of overweight and obesity, with a worrying acceleration of rates among children. In Germany, 10 and 6% of children and adolescents and more than 50 and 20% of the adult population are overweight and obese, respectively [1, 2]. The actual numbers in most of Europe are moving in the same direction [3].

Inverse Social Gradients in Overweight

In Western societies, there is an inverse social gradient in overweight; i.e. people from a low social class have the highest prevalence of overweight and obesity. Overweight is related to relative deprivation or one's position within a hierarchy. It is not confined to the poorest members of a society, but rather, the gradient in overweight is across the whole society. Since there are considerable differences among all social groups, the gradient suggests that overweight is not only a problem in one (i.e. the lowest) socio-economic status (SES) group. However, the increase in the prevalence of overweight that has been observed during the last 30 years is to a great part due to growth of the low-SES group [4, 5]. The SES gradient also suggests that overweight is an epiphenomenon reflecting problems in our societies as a whole; i.e. the varying quality of arrangements between groups in our societies.

The inverse social gradient in overweight is independent of age and sex. However, the steepest gradients in health have been observed in childhood and midlife, with lesser inequality in the elderly [6, 7]. In addition, there is an effect of gender in adults: the social gradient in health is steeper in adult men compared with women [6].

The onset of the social gradient has been investigated rarely [8]. At birth, a social gradient is already visible, but this gradient is positive, i.e. with increasing SES, birth weight increases. At the ages of 1 and 2 years, the SES gradient disappears. The inverse social gradient in overweight manifests between years 2 and 6 of life.

As shown by international studies, the social gradient in overweight has increased during the last 20 years [9, 10]. In Germany, SES gradients in overweight children have changed since 2005: the prevalence of overweight mostly increased in children of medium SES, reaching the values observed in the low-SES group [11]. Concomitantly, the prevalence of overweight remained nearly unchanged in the high- as well as the low-SES groups. Thus, regarding social inequality in overweight, there are only two different groups left: a high-SES group (with a relatively low prevalence of childhood overweight) and a 'low-plus-medium' SES group (with similar high numbers of overweight children).

Different Characteristics of Socio-Economic Status

Since SES is not a direct variable of overweight, which variable is the best proxy for SES must be questioned. In children, the highest parental education is mostly used. Other possibilities are income, completed vocational training, and living space (i.e. rooms per person). The inverse social gradient is independent of the proxy used, as low parental education, a parent without completed vocational training, low income, and a small living space are all nearly equally associated with the highest prevalence of overweight in children and adolescents [12].

Lifestyle, Overweight, and Socio-Economic Status

Lifestyle Factors and Overweight

Increasing body weight results from a positive energy balance and thus from lifestyle habits. A high intake of energy-dense foods, low physical activity, and high inactivity are considered to be the direct determinants of overweight, i.e. they all add to a positive energy balance. However, lifestyle variables have not shown consistent strong associations with either the prevalence or the incidence of overweight [13]. In most epidemiological studies, only inactivity (i.e. TV consumption), rather than physical activity, was found to be associated with overweight in children and adolescents [14]. Regarding food intake, soft drinks and fast-food consumption have been correlated with childhood and adolescent overweight [14, 15].

To summarize, lifestyle habits, as assessed by epidemiological methods or biomarkers, can partly explain overweight. Calculation of the attributable risks of overweight showed that 17.1% (relative) of overweight was attributable to media time; i.e. if all children and adolescents reduce their media time to <1 hour per day, the prevalence of overweight would decrease from 15 to 12.4% [16]. Longitudinal studies on the incidence of overweight in children and adolescents have argued in favor of only small imbalances in energy balance of 50 to 100 kcal/day [17]. These numbers are below the accuracy of present methods for the assessment of energy intake and/or energy expenditure, suggesting that the impact of lifestyle on overweight cannot be measured with confidence.

Lifestyle Factors and Socio-Economic Status

In fact, there are social gradients in food intake, activity, and inactivity [12, 18, 19]. The lower social status is, the higher the prevalence of unhealthy lifestyle habits in children and adolescents is. When compared with high-SES children, children from low-SES families consumed more soft drinks, fast food, and white bread and had lower intake of fruit and vegetables. Concomitantly, low-SES children had higher TV consumption. In addition, children of a low SES were less physically active.

Lifestyle Factors, Socio-Economic Status, and Overweight

It is likely that social inequalities in overweight in children partly depend on socially determined health behavior. Lifestyle factors can mediate the relationship between SES and BMI. In a study conducted in Germany and the US, in 10- to 17-year-old adolescents, the effect of SES on overweight was partially mediated by media exposure, which explained 35% of the SES-BMI association in the German sample and 16% in the US sample [20]. Besides this mediation effect, there was also a moderator effect of SES in the relationship between media time and overweight: an increased risk of overweight with increasing media consumption was obvious in children from families of middle or high SES [13]. By contrast, among low-SES individuals, the prevalence of overweight was independent of media time.

Migration Background

The impact of social determinants of health also becomes obvious in children of different ethnic affiliations. When compared with German children, the prevalence of overweight was higher in immigrant children living in Germany [1, 13]. However,

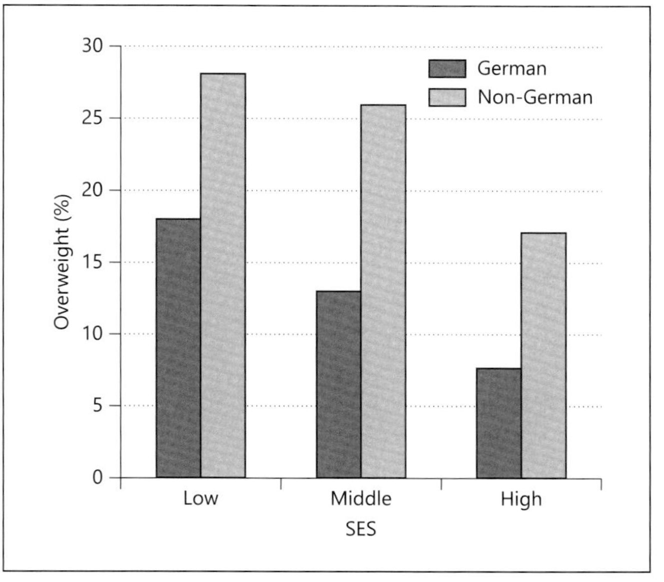

Fig. 1. Inverse social gradient in overweight in German and non-German children and adolescents.

even in this population, there was an inverse SES gradient in overweight (fig. 1). When compared with the inverse gradient in overweight obtained for German children, the inverse gradient in non-German immigrant children was shifted upward, with the prevalence of overweight nearly doubled in all SES groups [12].

Comparing lifestyle habits between German and non-German children living in Germany, differences were obvious among the various social groups [12]. While media consumption was considerably higher in non-German children in all SES groups, the prevalence of an unhealthy eating index was doubled in non-German children in the high-SES group only. Physical activity was the same between German and non-German children of low SES; however, middle- and high-SES German children were more often physically active than non-German children.

Social Environment and Overweight

Overweight distributes within social networks, which again determine values, behavior, norms about overweight, and self-esteem [21]. Unhealthy behaviors are supported by obesogenic environments, e.g. exposure to unhealthy food is higher in low-SES areas [22], driving children to over-consume certain foods (i.e. mostly energy-dense and high-fat foods). In addition, high traffic density and a high crime rate are associated with a longer media time. This is especially true for children from families with a low-SES background. Thus, unhealthy environments may be conducive to unhealthy living. Obesogenic environments together with restricted resources (e.g. education or money) disproportionally affect low-SES groups (fig. 2).

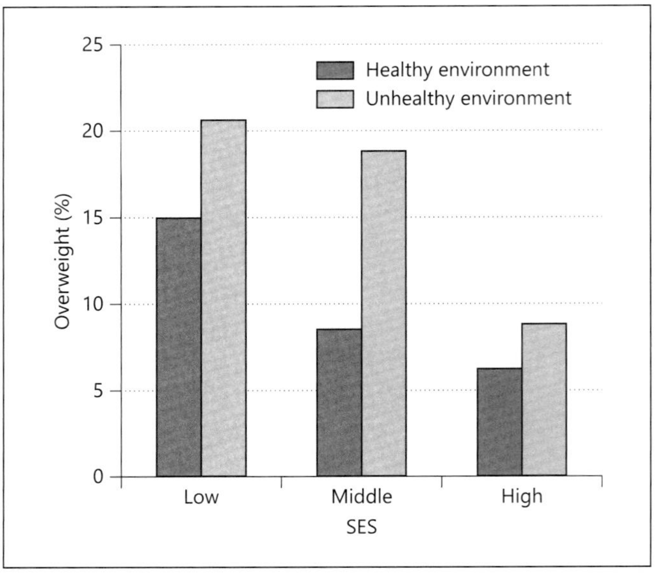

Fig. 2. Social gradient in overweight between children living in healthy and unhealthy environments. Healthy environment: districts with a low unemployment rate, a low proportion of immigrants, and a low percentage of welfare recipients. Unhealthy environment: districts with a high unemployment rate, a high proportion of immigrants, and a high percentage of welfare recipients.

Socio-Economic Status as a Barrier against Preventive Measures

SES also serves as a barrier against preventive measures. Socially selective effects of school-based programs for health promotion have been documented within follow-up periods of 4 and 8 years [23, 24]. Efficiency in terms of the prevalence and incidence of overweight differed between different social groups, and success was only observed among children from high-SES families. By contrast, no or even negative effects were seen in middle- or low-SES children.

Similar results have been obtained after family-based prevention of overweight. These programs were effective in children of high-SES families only [25]. By contrast, overweight children with a low-SES background increased, rather than decreased, in body weight after intervention.

Socio-economic differences in the outcomes of preventive measures are not explained by socio-economic differentials in knowledge [26]. For example, school-based intervention increased knowledge about nutrition in 6-year-old children, and the effect was independent of social position. Differences in health literacy, rather than knowledge, may add to social barriers against preventive measures [27].

Perspective

To understand population obesity (and also socio-economic gradients in obesity), we have to take into account further determinants of obesity, including the micro- and macro-environment, e.g. food production and supply, income inequality, education, culture, globalization, urbanization, transition, and westernization as well as political economy [28, 29]. Globalization may create opportunities that reduce poverty and improve health by diffusion of medical advances. By contrast, it also creates social contexts (i.e. it tends to reinforce the divergence of incomes and opportunities) that have negative effects on inequality in health and overweight.

References

1 Kurth BM, Schaffrath Rosario A: [Overweight and obesity in children and adolescents in Germany]. Bundesgesundheitsblatt Gesundheitsforschung Gesundheitsschutz 2010;53:643–652.

2 Mensink GB, Schienkiewitz A, Haftenberger M, et al: [Overweight and obesity in Germany: results of the German Health Interview and Examination Survey for Adults (DEGS1)]. Bundesgesundheitsblatt Gesundheitsforschung Gesundheitsschutz 2013;56:786–794.

3 Lobstein T, Baur L, Uauy R, et al: Obesity in children and young people: a crisis in public health. Obes Rev 2004;5(Suppl 1):4–104.

4 Molarius A, Seidell JC, Sans S, et al: Educational level, relative body weight, and changes in their association over 10 years: an international perspective from the WHO MONICA project. Am J Public Health 2000;90:1260–1268.

5 Stamatakis E, Primatesta P, Chinn S, et al: Overweight and obesity trends from 1974 to 2003 in English children: what is the role of socioeconomic factors? Arch Dis Child 2005;90:999–1004.

6 Siegrist J, Marmot M: Social inequalities in health: basic facts. in Siegrist J, Marmot M (eds) Social Inequalities in Health: New Evidence and Practice Implications. Oxford, Oxford University Press, 2006.

7 Giskes K, van Lenthe FJ, Turrell G, et al: Socioeconomic position at different stages of the life course and its influence on body weight and weight gain in adulthood: A longitudinal study with 13-year follow-up. Obesity (Silver Spring) 2008;16:1377–1381.

8 Langnäse K, Mast M, Danielzik S, et al: Socioeconomic gradients in body weight of German children reverse direction between the ages of 2 and 6 years. J Nutr 2003;133:789–796.

9 Stamatakis E, Wardle J, Cole TJ: Childhood obesity and overweight prevalence trends in England: evidence for growing socioeconomic disparities. Int J Obes (Lond) 2010;34:41–47.

10 Wang Y, Zhang Q: Are American children and adolescents of low socioeconomic status at increased risk of obesity? Changes in the association between overweight and family income between 1971 and 2002. Am J Clin Nutr 2006;84:707–716.

11 Johannsen M: Übergewicht bei 5- bis 7-jährigen Kindern – analyse von trends, Determinanten und gesundheitlichen Auswirkungen. Eine Untersuchung im Rahmen der Kieler Adipositas-Präventionsstudie (KOPS), dissertation, Christian-Albrechts-Universität zu Kiel, Kiel, 2009.

12 Lange D, Plachta-Danielzik S, Landsberg B, et al: [Social inequality, migration, and healthy environments as determinants of overweight of children and adolescents. Results of the Kiel Obesity Prevention Study (KOPS)]. Bundesgesundheitsblatt Gesundheitsforschung Gesundheitsschutz 2010;53:707–715.

13 Plachta-Danielzik S, Landsberg B, Johannsen M, et al: Determinants of the prevalence and incidence of overweight in children and adolescents. Public Health Nutr 2010;13:1870–1881.

14 Must A, Barish EE, Bandini LG: Modifiable risk factors in relation to changes in BMI and fatness: what have we learned from prospective studies of school-aged children? Int J Obes (Lond) 2009;33:705–715.

15 Pereira MA, Kartashov AI, Ebbeling CB, et al: Fast-food habits, weight gain, and insulin resistance (the cardia study): 15-year prospective analysis. Lancet 2005;365:36–42.

16 Plachta-Danielzik S, Kehden B, Landsberg B, et al: Attributable risks for childhood overweight: evidence for limited effectiveness of prevention. Pediatrics 2012;130:e865–e871.

17 Plachta-Danielzik S, Landsberg B, Bosy-Westphal A, et al: Energy gain and energy gap in normal-weight children: longitudinal data of the KOPS. Obesity (Silver Spring) 2008;16:777–783.

18 Danielzik S, Pust S, Landsberg B, et al: Sozio-ökonomische Einflüsse auf gesundheit und Übergewicht. Ernährungs Umschau Int 2006;6:212–2017.

19 Langnäse K, Mast M, Müller MJ: Social class differences in overweight of prepubertal children in northwest Germany. Int J Obes Relat Metab Disord 2002;26:566–572.

20 Morgenstern M, Sargent JD, Hanewinkel R: Relation between socioeconomic status and body mass index: evidence of an indirect path via television use. Arch Pediatr Adolesc Med 2009;163:731–738.

21 Christakis NA, Fowler JH: The spread of obesity in a large social network over 32 years. N Engl J Med 2007;357:370–379.
22 Lange D: Einfluss von Sozialen Faktoren und der Lebenswelten auf den Ernährungszustand und Lebensstil von Kindern und Jugendlichen der Kieler Adipoitas-Präventionsstudie (KOPS); dissertation, Schriftenreihe des Instituts für Humanernährung und Lebensmittelkunde der Christian-Albrechts-Universität zu Kiel, Kiel, 2009.
23 Plachta-Danielzik S, Landsberg B, Lange D, et al: Eight-year follow-up of school-based intervention on childhood overweight – the Kiel Obesity Prevention Study. Obes Facts 2011;4:35–43.
24 Plachta-Danielzik S, Pust S, Asbeck I, et al: Four-year follow-up of school-based intervention on overweight children: the KOPS study. Obesity (Silver Spring) 2007;15:3159–3169.
25 Langnäse K, Asbeck I, Mast M, et al: Influence of socio-economic status on the long-term effect of family-based intervention in prepubertal overweight children. Health Educ 2004;104:336–343.
26 Danielzik S, Pust S, Müller MJ: School-based interventions to prevent overweight and obesity in prepubertal children: process and 4-years outcome evaluation of the Kiel Obesity Prevention Study (KOPS). Acta Paediatr Suppl 2007;96:19–25.
27 Schmidt CO, Fahland RA, Franze M, et al: Health-related behaviour, knowledge, attitudes, communication and social status in school children in eastern Germany. Health Educ Res 2010;25:542–551.
28 Gortmaker SL, Swinburn BA, Levy D, et al: Changing the future of obesity: science, policy, and action. Lancet 2011;378:838–847.
29 Müller MJ: How are we going to turn the obesity prevention experience? Obes Rev 2010;11:101–104.

Prof. Dr. Manfred James Müller
Institut für Humanernährung und Lebensmittelkunde
Christian-Albrechts-Universität zu Kiel
Düsternbrooker Weg 17
DE–24105 Kiel (Germany)
E-Mail mmueller@nutrfoodsc.uni-kiel.de

Kiess W, Wabitsch M, Maffeis C, Sharma AM (eds): Metabolic Syndrome and Obesity in Childhood and Adolescence.
Pediatr Adolesc Med. Basel, Karger, 2015, vol 19, pp 75–83 (DOI: 10.1159/000368108)

Carbohydrate Metabolism

Martin Wabitsch · Christian Denzer

Interdisciplinary Obesity Unit, Division of Pediatric Endocrinology and Diabetes, Department of Pediatrics and Adolescent Medicine, University Medical Center Ulm, University of Ulm, Ulm, Germany

Abstract

The central pathogenetic feature of the metabolic syndrome is insulin resistance. The term 'insulin resistance' refers to reduced glucose uptake in the whole body in response to physiological insulin levels. The progression from normal glucose tolerance to impaired glucose tolerance accompanies decreasing insulin sensitivity and increasing insulin resistance. This chapter provides insight into the molecular basis and the pathophysiology of the regulation of insulin sensitivity and resistance. In this respect, the role of increased adipose tissue and ectopic adipose tissue in relation to insulin resistance is highlighted.

Type 2 Diabetes in Children and Adolescents

Changes in lifestyle resulting in changes in food consumption and exercise are responsible for the worldwide increase in obesity. Until recently, type 2 diabetes mellitus had been a rare condition in children and adolescents (fig. 1). Since the mid-1990s, an increasing prevalence of type 2 diabetes in children and adolescents has been reported, in parallel to an increase in obesity. In some ethnic populations, type 2 diabetes is now the predominant form of diabetes in adolescents in the United States.

The clinical and metabolic presentation of type 2 diabetes mellitus in Caucasian adolescents differs from that in Afro-Americans, Mexicans, Hispanics, or Native Americans. In these ethnic groups, up to 25% of children with suspected type 2 diabetes present with ketoacidosis, whereas diabetic ketoacidosis is a rare event in Caucasian adolescents with type 2 diabetes. Overt clinical signs or symptoms of diabetes are rarely present in this group, and acanthosis nigricans is absent in 50% of patients. These differences may be explained by the fact that most of these cases are detected by screening programs, in contrast to published data from non-Caucasian populations, which are reported in case series of patients with overt clinical symptoms.

As in adults, undiagnosed type 2 diabetes mellitus is a common condition in obese children and adolescents. Therefore, screening for type 2 diabetes in children and

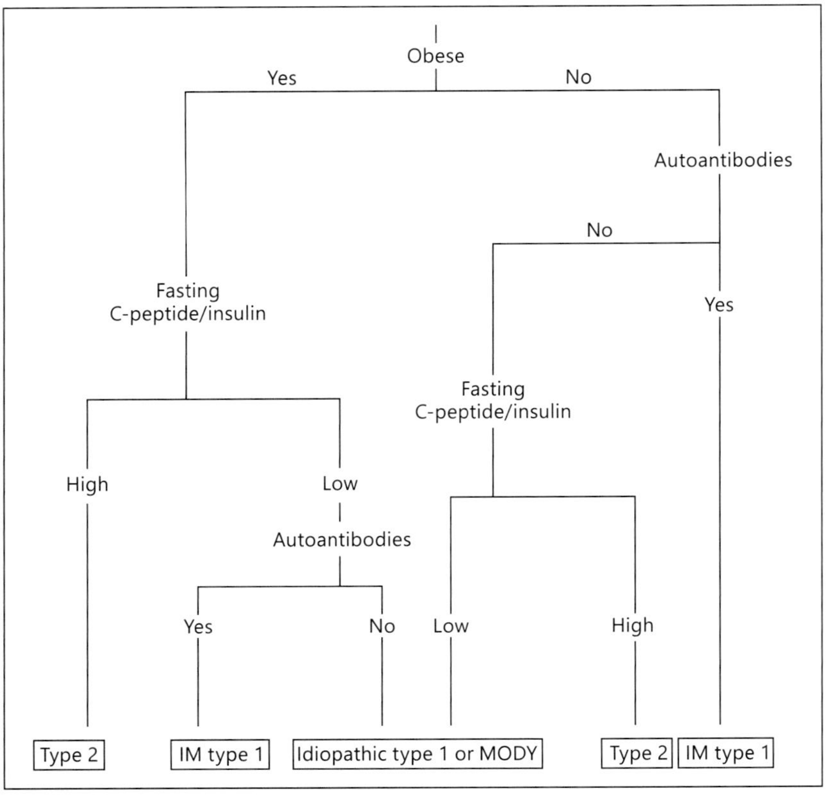

Fig. 1. Flowchart for the classification of diabetes mellitus in children and adolescents, adapted from the recommendations of the American Diabetes Association [5].

adolescents with obesity is recommended. Unrecognized hyperglycemia will contribute to both microvascular and macrovascular risks in later life. A recent German screening study demonstrated a prevalence rate of type 2 diabetes of approximately 1% in obese Caucasian children and adolescents [1].

As proposed by the American Diabetes Association, screening for type 2 diabetes in Caucasian children and adolescents should be initiated from age 10 or at the onset of puberty (whichever comes first) in high-risk patients, who either have a family history of type 2 diabetes in first- and second-degree relatives or present with clinical signs of insulin resistance or impaired glucose homeostasis (i.e. acanthosis nigricans) or with comorbid conditions associated with insulin resistance (i.e. hypertension, dyslipidemia). Screening for diabetes should also be performed in all extremely obese children and adolescents.

Studies using HbA1c as a screening tool were disappointing, since one third of asymptomatic children with type 2 diabetes mellitus demonstrated normal values. Studies testing the applicability of HbA1c after its standardization as a screening tool are lacking to date.

Glucose Homeostasis in Obese Children and Adolescents

The progression from normal glucose tolerance to impaired glucose tolerance (IGT) accompanies decreasing insulin sensitivity and increasing insulin resistance. IGT is an intermediate stage before the development of diabetes. Puberty is a major factor influencing glucose tolerance in children and adolescents. Euglycemic-hyperinsulinemic clamp studies demonstrated that insulin-mediated glucose disposal is 30% lower on average in adolescents at Tanner stages II, III, and IV compared with either prepubertal children or young adults. The observed differences in insulin sensitivity are partly caused by the increased secretion of growth hormone during puberty. Interestingly, there is a high spontaneous conversion rate from IGT to normal glucose tolerance during an observation period of 3–5 years in children and adolescents. This might be due to a reduction in insulin resistance in the last period of pubertal development.

Insulin Resistance and Glucose Regulation

Determination of the fasting serum insulin concentration allows calculation of insulin resistance indices (e.g. the homeostasis model assessment of insulin resistance or quantitative insulin sensitivity check index). However, the main component of all of these indices is the fasting serum insulin concentration, which is characterized by high intraindividual physiological variability. Therefore, the significance of insulin resistance or insulin sensitivity indices calculated from fasting samples alone is questionable, and routine use of these indices in clinical settings for the evaluation of glucose homeostasis in individual subjects cannot be recommended. It must also be noted that the analytic methodology of insulin measurement is not yet standardized. The gold standard for the measurement of insulin resistance is the euglycemic-hyperinsulinemic clamp, a time-consuming, invasive and expensive method that is reserved for scientific research settings.

Insulin Resistance as the Central Pathomechanism of the Metabolic Syndrome

The central pathogenetic feature of the metabolic syndrome (MetS) is insulin resistance. The term 'insulin resistance' refers to reduced glucose uptake in the whole body in response to physiological insulin levels. Euglycemic-hyperinsulinemic clamp studies revealed that whole-body insulin sensitivity/insulin resistance is mainly determined by insulin-mediated glucose disposal at the level of the skeletal muscle (>75% of the amount of glucose during the clamp study is absorbed by the muscle, and 2–3% is absorbed by adipose tissue). Nevertheless, adipose tissue itself, the distribution of adipose tissue, and the partitioning of lipids in different tissues have key roles in the regulation of glucose metabolism, especially with increasing fat mass (see below).

Convincing evidence from epidemiologic studies illustrates the importance of environmental factors during sensitive phases of fetal (and probably postnatal) development for an individual's metabolic phenotype not only in childhood and adolescence but also in adulthood (the concept of 'fetal programming', or the Barker hypothesis). Children who were born to mothers with poorly controlled diabetes and children born small for gestational age who experience rapid catch-up weight gain during infancy develop a marked phenotype of insulin resistance in later life. These unfavorable metabolic changes are most likely mediated by epigenetic mechanisms.

In pediatrics and adolescent medicine, is it important to note that during adolescence, physiological insulin resistance is observed in the body. During adolescence, there is a 25–50% decrease in the insulin sensitivity of the body, which returns to normal after the end of adolescence.

The Molecular Basis of Insulin Resistance in the Metabolic Syndrome

Insulin mediates its effect on target tissues via specific membrane receptors [2]. The insulin receptor consists of an extracellular α-subunit and two transmembrane β-subunits, which are linked by disulfide bonds. The binding of insulin to the α-subunit results in a change in the three-dimensional receptor structure (conformation), which causes autophosphorylation of the β-subunit. Receptor activation leads to the phosphorylation of insulin receptor substrate proteins, which are in turn coupled to another kinase, or phosphoinositide-3-kinase. This lipid kinase phosphorylates the signal transducer phosphatidylinositol bisphosphate to phosphatidylinositol triphosphate, which ultimately activates the central kinase of the insulin signaling pathway, Akt. The insulin signal is now passed on to the various effector pathways. Thus, uptake of glucose into the cell through glucose transporter-4 or synthesis of glycogen is activated. Insulin stimulates glycogen synthesis and inhibits hepatic gluconeogenesis and glycogenolysis (fig. 2).

In the MetS – or 'insulin resistance syndrome' – the number of insulin receptors is reduced. This down-regulation is triggered by the existing hyperinsulinemia. Moreover, the tyrosine kinase activity of the insulin receptor is lowered, resulting in a further disturbance of proximal signal transmission.

Insulin is an anabolic hormone and thus a negative regulator of β-adrenergic-stimulated lipolysis [2]. With insulin resistance, there is reduced insulin-mediated inhibition of basal lipolysis. Together with increased body fat mass, this contributes to an increase in the level of circulating free fatty acids (FFAs). FFAs are in turn causally related to insulin resistance and reactive hyperinsulinemia in three different ways. FFAs reduce insulin binding to its receptor and decrease –

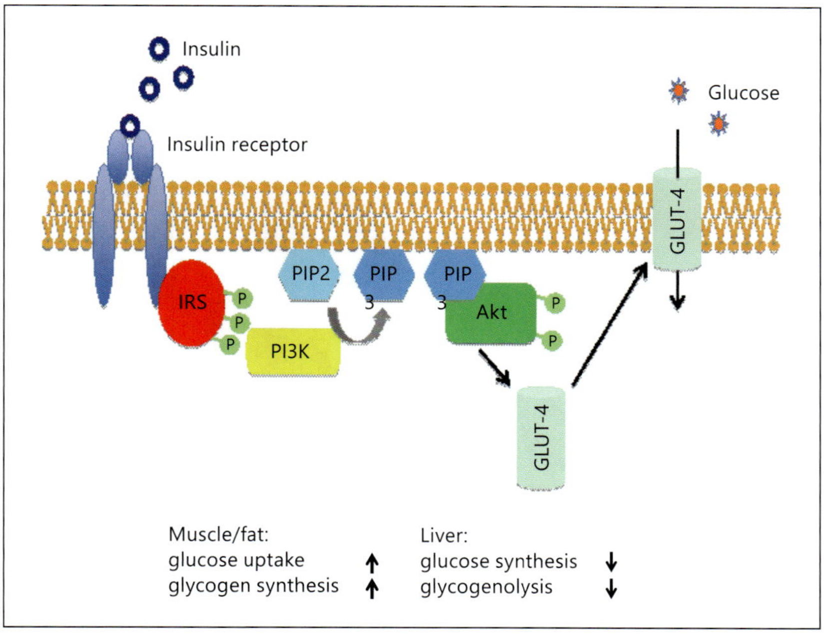

Fig. 2. Insulin-mediated signal transmission [4]. Insulin binds to the extracellular α-subunit of the insulin receptor. This leads to the autophosphorylation of the intracellular β-subunit of the receptor and to additional phosphorylation of insulin receptor substrate (IRS) proteins. This in turn results in the activation of phosphoinositide 3-kinase (PI3K), which catalyzes the conversion of phosphatidylinositol diphosphate (PIP2) to phosphatidylinositol triphosphate (PIP3). The lipid molecule activates the key kinase Akt, which then forwards the insulin signal to the various cell effector systems. In adipose tissue as well as in the muscle, glucose transporter-4 (GLUT-4) is translocated to the cell surface, and glucose is imported into the cell. Glycogen synthesis is stimulated, whereas hepatic gluconeogenesis and glycogenolysis are inhibited by insulin.

depending on the concentration – insulin clearance in the liver. Furthermore, glucose utilization in the muscle is significantly impaired by high levels of FFAs. FFAs inhibit the tyrosine phosphorylation of insulin receptor substrate-1, which results in a reduced activity of phosphoinositide-3-kinase and impaired glucose uptake. The resulting discrete hyperglycemia causes permanent stimulation of insulin secretion, with the consequence of hyperinsulinemia. Adding to the state of chronic hyperinsulinemia, high levels of FFAs directly stimulate insulin secretion by the β-cells.

The Role of Adipose Tissue in the Pathogenesis of Insulin Resistance and the Metabolic Syndrome

Core components of the MetS, or hypertension, dyslipidemia and insulin resistance, are closely associated with the degree of obesity and with body fat mass.

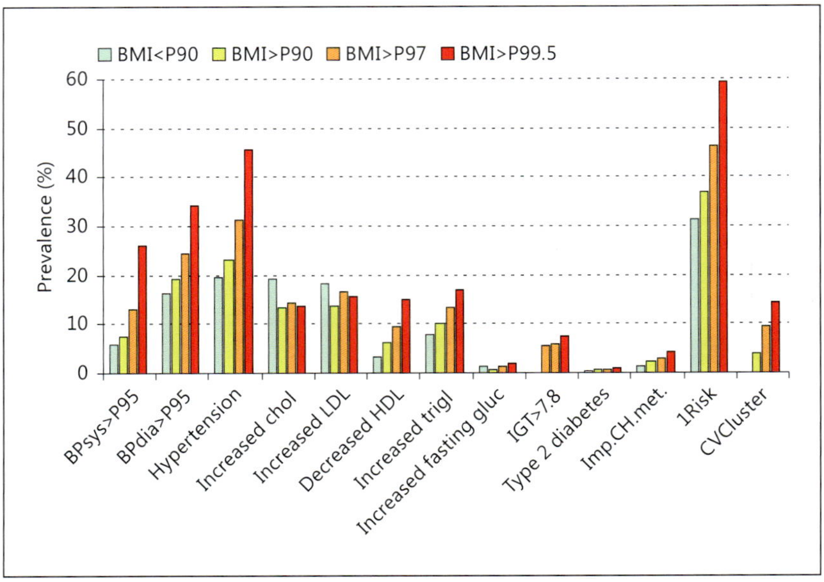

Fig. 3. Cardiovascular risk factors in relation to body mass index (BMI) categories in 26,008 overweight children and adolescents (an analysis of the APV registry) [6]. BP = blood pressure; P = percentile; IGT = impaired glucose tolerance (>7.8 mmol/l after a 2 h oral glucose tolerance test); DM2 = diabetes mellitus type 2, defined by an impaired fasting glucose (IFG) >7 and/or a 2 h oral glucose tolerance test result >11.1 mmol/l; CH = carbohydrate; CVCluster = two or three cardiovascular clusters; 1Risk = risk of accumulation of two or more cardiovascular risk factors; BPdia = diastolic BP; BPsys = systolic BP; chol = cholesterol; fasting gluc = fasting glucose; HDL = high-density lipoprotein; Imp.CH.met. = impaired CH metabolism; LDL = low-density lipoprotein; trigl = triglyceride.

An analysis of 26,000 datasets from children and adolescents from the German obesity patient registry APV demonstrated that an increasing relative body mass index is directly associated with an increasing number of traditional cardiovascular risk factors, with a clear trend toward a clustering of these risk factors with increasing obesity (fig. 3).

This clear association of the degree of obesity and the manifestation of individual components of the MetS implies a causal relationship between increased fat mass and adverse metabolic changes (fig. 4). Recent studies have shown that adipose tissue mass, and particularly visceral fat mass, contributes to the development of insulin resistance as well as to the development of dyslipidemia and impaired β-cell function [3]. Increased levels of circulating fatty acids released from the visceral fat depot pass through the portal vein to the liver, acting as a substrate for the endogenous synthesis of very-low-density lipoproteins, which are in turn increasingly secreted by the liver. The increased supply of glycerol and lactate in the portal circulation leads to increased gluconeogenesis and hepatic glucose production as a result of substrate pressure.

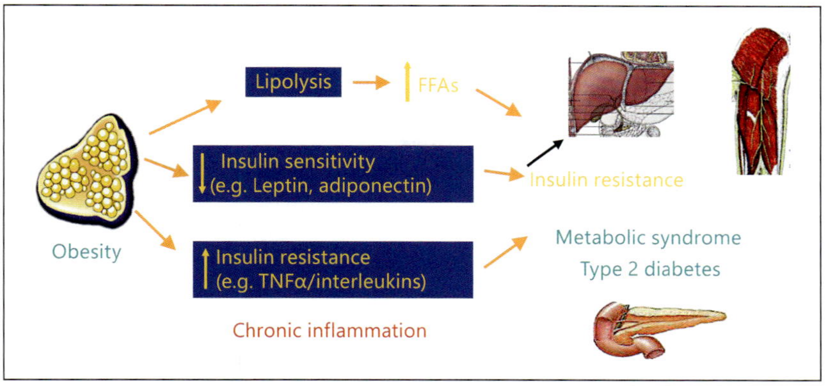

Fig. 4. The role of adipose tissue in the pathogenesis of insulin resistance and the metabolic syndrome.

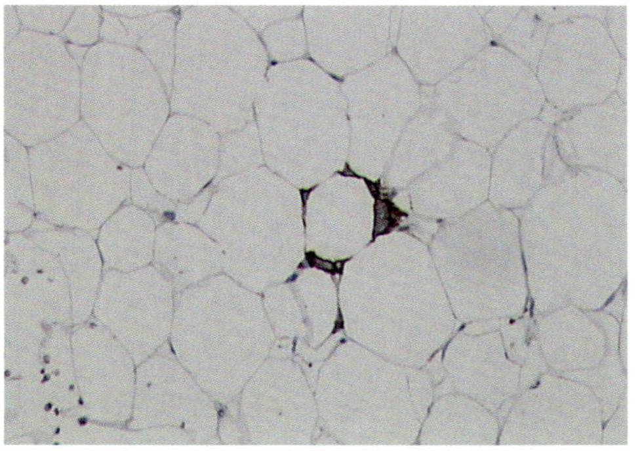

Fig. 5. Obesity-associated inflammation of adipose tissue. In obesity, macrophages migrate into the adipose tissue. In the figure, CD11c-positive macrophages are visible in the visceral adipose tissue of an obese patient. Macrophages surround a fat cell and form a crown-like structure. This inflammation of adipose tissue plays an important role in the pathogenesis of obesity-associated insulin resistance.

Figure 4 shows the relationship between increased fat mass and insulin resistance, involving dysfunction of glucose regulation via impaired β-cell function.

Adipose tissue secretes a wealth of adipokines, many of which interfere with the regulation of glucose homeostasis. Visceral adipose tissue produces relatively large amounts of insulin resistance-promoting adipokines. In addition to the effect of increased FFA levels, these adipokines enhance hepatic insulin resistance and counteract insulin's suppressive effect on hepatic gluconeogenesis, impair peripheral glucose uptake in the skeletal muscle and possibly impair β-cell function.

A pathognomonic feature of obesity-associated insulin resistance is chronic inflammation of the adipose tissue. Histopathologically, macrophages accumulate in adipose tissue and surround adipocytes in crown-like structures (fig. 5). Furthermore, genes involved in inflammatory pathways are overexpressed in macrophage-infiltrated adipose tissue. These hallmark changes in adipose tissue can be observed very early in the course of obesity and the development of obesity-related comorbidity, i.e. before a significant increase in the circulating insulin concentration, and must therefore be considered an early pathophysiological event in the development of the MetS.

Ectopic Fat Storage in the Muscle and Liver

Numerous experimental results support the idea that adipose tissue may reach its capacity limits as a fat storage depot in obesity. In this scenario, the adipose tissue is characterized by hypertrophy of the adipocyte. The hypertrophic adipocytes are insulin resistant and typically produce high levels of insulin resistance-promoting adipokines. Interestingly, individuals with insulin resistance show ectopic fat accumulation in the muscle and liver, probably due to having exceeded the capacity of the adipose tissue. Histologic fat measurements in muscle and liver biopsies, as well as measurements of intracellular lipid content by magnetic resonance spectroscopy, demonstrate markedly increased intramyocellular and intrahepatocellular triglyceride concentrations in patients with the MetS. An increased intramyocellular lipid concentration is closely and inversely correlated to whole-body insulin sensitivity. The accumulation of intramyocellular fat is triggered by reduced fat oxidation in the state of insulin resistance as well as by increased availability of fatty acids because of impaired suppression of lipolysis in adipose tissue. There is also a direct link between visceral fat mass and the occurrence of nonalcoholic steatohepatitis, namely, fat accumulation in hepatocytes. The findings of fat accumulation in the skeletal muscle and liver are typical in patients in whom the MetS is present.

In this context, it is interesting to note that patients without or with reduced adipose tissue (e.g. with connatal or acquired lipodystrophy), a disease state in which the maximum storage capacity of adipose tissue is extremely restricted, are affected by similar adverse metabolic changes as obese patients with the MetS. As in patients with obesity and the MetS, in patients with lipodystrophies, there is also an accumulation of fat in the skeletal muscle and in the liver. According to these findings, functionally healthy adipose tissue, which is characterized by high insulin sensitivity and a high storage capacity, is essential for a healthy metabolism and helps to prevent the development of the MetS.

The Effects of Lifestyle Interventions

Exercise and physical activity have a positive effect on insulin sensitivity and on proinflammatory activity (e.g. reduction of serum interleukin-6 concentrations), as well as on body weight development and maintenance after body weight reduction. Lifestyle intervention programs have been found to be more effective and more efficient than pharmacotherapy for the prevention of progression from IGT to overt type 2 diabetes in obese adults. The same is probably true for children and adolescents. Long-term treatment of obesity, probably including extended pharmacotherapy, may be necessary for adolescents with extreme obesity, since diet and exercise programs alone and in combination with educational interventions have been proven to fail in the majority of cases in the long term. For specific treatment strategies for children and adolescents with obesity, please refer to chapter 4.

Acknowledgments

The authors thank Bettina Wabitsch for expert secretarial assistance. This chapter was written based on an article in German in the Journal of the Germany Society for Pediatrics and Adolescent Medicine [4].

References

1 Wabitsch M, Hauner H, Hertrampf M, et al: Type II diabetes mellitus and impaired glucose regulation in Caucasian children and adolescents with obesity living in Germany. Int J Obes Relat Metab Disord 2004; 28:307–313.
2 Saltiel AR, Kahn CR: Insulin signalling and the regulation of glucose and lipid metabolism. Nature 2001; 414:799–806.
3 Wirth A, Hauner H, Jacob S: Metabolisches Syndrom und Insulinresistenz: Ätiologie und Mechanismen; in Wirth A (ed): Das Metabolische Syndrom. München, Urban & Vogel, 2007, pp 56–80.
4 Wabitsch M, Moss A, Denzer C, et al: Das metabolische Syndrom. Monatsschr Kinderheilkd 2012; 160:277–292.
5 American Diabetes Association: Type 2 diabetes in children and adolescents. American Diabetes Association. Diabetes Care 2000; 23:381–389.
6 I'Allemand D, Wiegand S, Reinehr T, et al: Cardiovascular risk in 26,008 European overweight children as established by a multicenter database. Obesity 2008; 16:1672–1679.

Martin Wabitsch, MD, PhD
Interdisciplinary Obesity Unit, Division of Pediatric Endocrinology and Diabetes
Department of Pediatrics and Adolescent Medicine
University Medical Center Ulm, University of Ulm
Eythstrasse 24, DE–89075 Ulm (Germany)
E-Mail martin.wabitsch@uniklinik-ulm.de

Kiess W, Wabitsch M, Maffeis C, Sharma AM (eds): Metabolic Syndrome and Obesity in Childhood and Adolescence.
Pediatr Adolesc Med. Basel, Karger, 2015, vol 19, pp 84–98 (DOI: 10.1159/000368110)

Orthopaedic Aspects of Obesity in Children and Adults

Falk Thielemann · Klaus-Peter Guenther · Maik Stiehler

University Centre of Orthopaedics and Traumatology, University Hospital Carl Gustav Carus at Technical University Dresden, Dresden, Germany

Abstract

Obese patients often complain of pain in their postural and locomotor apparatus. Besides functional disabilities resulting from increased soft tissue on the trunk and extremities, malalignment and structural changes in the load-bearing joints of the lower extremities and spine are mainly responsible for this complaint. It has been clearly documented that in children and adolescents, there is a relationship between the development of pathological foot, knee and hip disorders as well as leg axis malalignment and the early manifestation of overweight or even obesity. Accident statistics have revealed an increased risk of injury in overweight children and adolescents during everyday life and sporting activities. The determination of an optimal obesity treatment for the prevention of diseases and the resulting damage to the musculoskeletal system described below is thus of central importance.

Foot Deformities

The tarsal skeleton of the adult has a medially open arch-shaped form that is supported by strong plantar foot ligaments, the plantar fascia and the intrinsic foot muscles. These structures enable the absorption of the pressure load during the stance phase and spring from the body in an elastic way at the beginning of the swing phase. The active and passive arch structures reach their full efficiencies over the course of a child's growth. Basically, a mild planovalgus foot with a slightly flattened longitudinal arch is a physiological finding during infancy and adulthood that has no significant pathological value. While standing and walking, a mild deformity can be actively compensated for into old age by the inverter extrinsic muscles, particularly

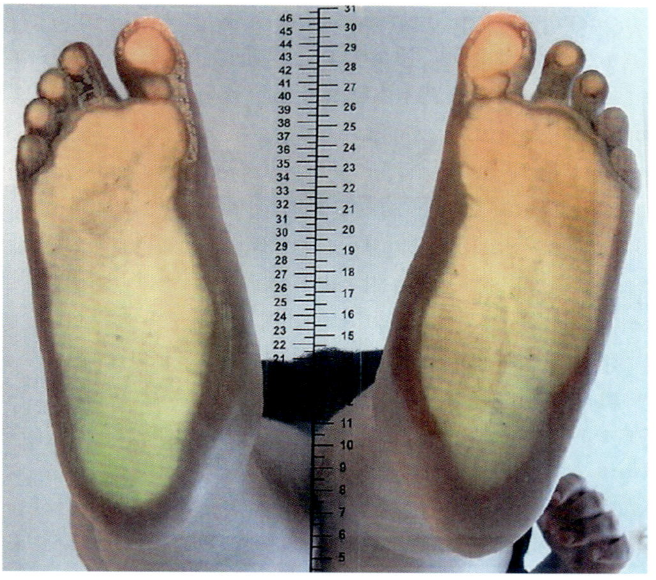

Fig. 1. Podogram of an overweight 12-year-old boy with bilateral flexible flatfeet (BMI 27.3). The plantar loading area is completely medially shifted. The notch on the medial border of the foot, i.e. the longitudinal arch, does not exist in either foot.

the posterior tibial muscle. The active muscular and passive ligament compensatory capacities are limited. Besides constitutional ligament weakness, early onset and long-term overweight represent essential links to the possible decompensation of the sub- and pretalar arch structures and thus to the dynamic shock-absorbing function of the feet. In cases of pronounced instability of the tarsal joint complex, under load-bearing conditions, there is pronation-abduction of the subtalar joint complex. Although there is no universally accepted definition of flatfoot, the following clinical and anatomical characteristics are typical features of this deformity during the stance phase:

- hindfoot valgus: pronounced hindfoot eversion of the subtalar complex
- prominence of the talar head at the medioplantar load area: medioplantar subluxation of the talus in the talocalcaneal joint
- forefoot abduction: dorsiflexion and abduction of the navicular and cuboid bones (Chopart's joint series).

Besides the inability to withstand load bearing during daily life activities, affected children and adults complain of diffuse discomfort in the feet and also frequently throughout the entire musculoskeletal system.

In these individuals, the static footprint while standing shows the absence of the notch on the plantar surface exposed to stresses in the middle of the medial border and thus the loss of the longitudinal arch of the foot (fig. 1). In severe cases, flatfoot may even result in the loss of contact of the lateral column with complete medial displacement of the plantar surface. In these cases, there is often medioplantar callus formation at the level of the dislocated talar head or even skin ulcers that develop due to the pathological patterns of plantar pressure.

Impact of Obesity on the Paediatric Foot

In a previous study, Horn [1] has drawn attention to the increased clinical prevalence of flatfoot in obese children (body mass index [BMI] >30), suggesting a relationship between infantile obesity and its occurrence. In a number of scientific studies, attempts have been made to examine the influence of overweight and obesity on the growing foot. Based on the static footprints of 431 prepubescent Australian children, Riddiford-Harland et al. [2] were able to show significant differences in plantar pressure patterns between obese and non-obese children. Dowling et al. [3, 4] published several studies on the effects of obesity on plantar pressure distribution patterns in prepubescent children. Measurements of static and dynamic foot pressure in children with overt obesity (mean ± standard deviation BMI 25.8 ± 3.8) compared to a control group of non-obese children of the same age (BMI 16.8 ± 2) were evaluated. Calculations of force and pressure distributions under loaded and unloaded conditions revealed interesting differences between the obese and non-obese children in terms of gait as well as static and dynamic stresses on the fore- and hindfoot. The authors postulated that discomfort and/or structural pathologies are associated with a distribution pattern of increased plantar forefoot pressure, which over the medium term leads to a lowering of the medial border of the foot when walking.

Clinical Relevance of Flatfeet in Children and Adults

Depending on their durations, overweight and obesity are important potential risk factors for the early decompensation of tarsal joint structures. Studies on the natural course of flatfoot deformity and the resultant foot problems in adulthood are scarce. Bruckner and Rosler [5] published a cross-sectional study of foot problems and relevant orthopaedic alterations in a cohort of 103 women. They underlined the relationship between the development of painful foot deformities and the presence of obesity. In particular, they reported a correlation of the development of a forefoot deformity with the loss of the transverse arch and formation of a bunion (hallux abducto valgus deformity) with increased body weight. Mertz and Mertz [6] described obesity as an important link between hyperuricaemia or gout and metatarsophalangeal joint osteoarthritis (OA) or hallux rigidus. They postulated that the accelerated emergence of this special form of OA is caused by obesity.

Diabetic Foot Syndrome

Overweight and obesity are often the result of a carbohydrate-rich diet. This, in particular, increases the risk of type 2 diabetes. Depending on the length of time elapsed with poorly controlled diabetes mellitus, there is an increased risk of diabetes-associated foot problems. The following changes are of pathological significance for the diabetic foot:

- diabetic macroangiopathy
- diabetic microangiopathy
- diabetic neuropathy

- diabetic osteoarthropathy
- diabetic fatty tissue atrophy
- diabetic myatrophy.

Changes in sensation in the feet and disorders of sweating and circulation lead to calluses, pressure ulcers, chronic soft-tissue bacterial and fungal infections and bone infections and even to diabetic gangrene. Epidemiological data suggest that approximately 40–75% of non-traumatic amputations can be attributed to diabetes-associated diseases. For this reason, the care of this very difficult group of patients can be successful only in the context of a closely coordinated interdisciplinary team approach. The integration of the patient into a well-organised outpatient foot clinic is desirable. In addition to the optimal management of this metabolic disorder by an internist, patients need specialised support with foot and shoe care, dietary counselling, and depending on the risk group that the patients belong to, access to specialised surgical disciplines.

Summary

Obesity can have a negative influence both on the physiological alignment of the longitudinal arch in the planovalgus foot during childhood and on the emergence of adult deformities and joint arthritis in the midfoot and forefoot. Overweight and obesity are often associated with metabolic disorders. Diabetes mellitus and its consequences represent a challenge in the care of patients with diabetic foot ulcers; the management of this group of patients cannot be accomplished without close interdisciplinary cooperation.

Angular Deformities of the Leg

Physiological Development of the Leg Axes and the Influence of Articular Load Bearing

During the growth phase, the healthy growth plates of long bones have the capacity to compensate for stress caused by bending, i.e. unilateral pressure loads caused by appositional growth. This results in a typical shape alteration in children and adolescents. Axes and torsions in the thigh, lower leg and foot undergo characteristic changes from infancy to childhood and adulthood, which influence each other. The varus alignment (bow legs) dominates in children beginning to adopt an upright position. At approximately 4–8 years of age, there is a slight overcorrection towards a valgus knee (knock-knees), and finally, after closure of the growth plates, physiological orientation takes place. The mechanical loading axis as the key indicator for the alignment of the load-bearing lower extremities should, from this time point on, run from the static centre of the femoral head through the centre of the knee joint down to the centre of the ankle (the so-called Mikulicz line). This orthograde orientation of the stress axis is an important prerequisite for life-long mobility without overload and the subsequent degeneration of all joints of the lower extremities.

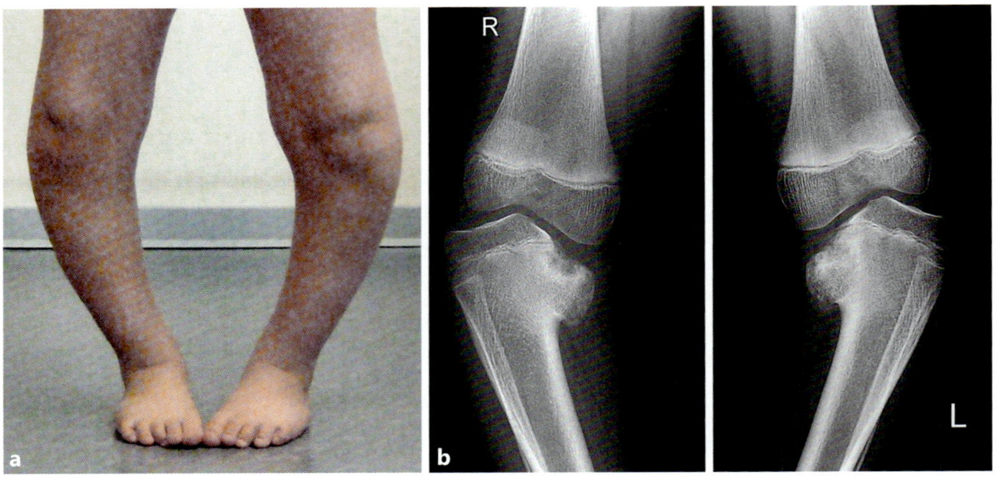

Fig. 2. Marked bilateral tibia vara with aseptic necrosis of the medial aspect of the tibial epiphysis in a 6-year-old girl with early manifestation of obesity. Clinical (**a**) and radiological (**b**) picture.

To determine whether a situation is pathological in a child or can still be considered as falling within the normal range, knowledge of the normal development of axes and torsions is essential.

According to Hefti [7], pathological forms of angular deformities in children and adolescents are rare. They may be congenital, post-traumatic, post-infectious and also present in metabolic diseases. Whether and to what extent the presence of obesity during the different stages of development of a child contributes to the persistence of the initial physiological conditions of the axis present in childhood or even to progression towards pathological alterations will be discussed below.

Tibia Vara (Morbus Blount) and Genu Varum

Idiopathic tibia vara, which is also termed osteochondrosis deformans tibiae or Morbus Blount [8], was first described and named by Blount and belongs to a group of aseptic osteochondronecrosis diseases. The disease is characterised by growth disturbance in the region of the medial aspect of the proximal tibial metaphysis and the epiphysis, which can lead to a progressive bow-leg deformity (genu varum).

Aetiology and Pathomechanism of Tibia Vara

Presumably, a combination of biological and mechanical factors (overload) leads to the deformation of the medial aspect of the proximal tibial epiphysis (fig. 2). Because this is frequently observed in Afro-Americans, a genetic predisposition to this condition is suspected. Pre-existing varus axis alignment in the affected extremity together with overweight or excessive activity and rapid growth are regarded as predisposing factors. The persistence of physiological genua vara during early childhood is a conspicuous feature of Blount disease because it normally regresses over the course of growth.

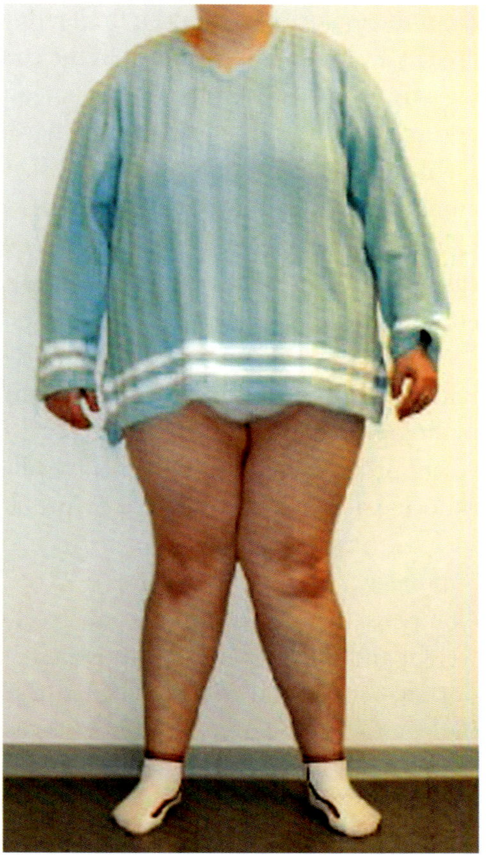

Fig. 3. Symptomatic bilateral genu valgum (knock-knees) in a 17-year-old obese adolescent.

Another interesting hypothesis on the aetiology of adolescent tibia vara has been proposed by Davids et al. [9]. In a biomechanical analysis, they investigated the hypothesis that an increased load on the medial knee compartment during the gait cycle can be a result of compensatory gait alterations in obese individuals with an enlarged thigh circumference ('fat-thigh gait'). With the help of three-dimensional gait analyses, different alterations, such as dynamic genu varum and increased knee rotation during the stance phase in addition to circumduction during the swing phase were identified. These pathological load cycles can create pressure stress in affected individuals, which can be sufficient to cause an alteration in the growth plate. The main differences between infant and adolescent tibia vara relate to the extent of the deformity and its tendency to recur after surgical correction as a consequence of the patient's age at the time of manifestation.

Genu Valgum

It should be noted that in overweight children and adults, varus misalignments are not exclusively observed. Clinically, valgus deformities (knock-knees) are more frequently present (fig. 3).

In the majority of children under 10 years of age, such a deformity can be considered as a variation of the norm in the context of the physiological development of the leg axis, which will undergo spontaneous correction over the course of growth. According to Hefti [7], this deformity hardly ever requires treatment.

In their investigation of musculoskeletal alterations in obese children with knee complaints, de Sá Pinto et al. [10], however, reported frequent valgus malalignments. Clinically, the extent of valgus leg axis deviations can be objectively determined quite easily by measuring the intermalleolar space. Values of >10 cm represent pathological conditions.

White et al. [11] underlined the need to distinguish between knock-knees presenting as a temporary stage during the physiological course of child development and pathological entities in relation to focal and systemic diseases. The latter entities represent progressive conditions that need to be treated, since pronounced genu valgum (knock-knees) represents a pre-arthrotic deformity.

Summary
Compensatory changes in the gait cycle and joint biomechanics accompanying overweight and the increase in soft tissue that occurs in children and adolescents are important aetiological links to the manifestation of severe growth-associated deviations in the axes of the lower extremities (tibia vara, genu varum and genu valgum).

Slipped Capital Femoral Epiphysis

A particularly severe hip disease in infants and adolescents is juvenile epiphysiolysis of the femoral neck growth plate. Because it involves a deformity that develops at the junction of the femoral head and femoral neck in association with a high risk of femoroacetabular impingement, this disease is deemed an essential cause of secondary hip OA.

Frequency
Slipped capital femoral epiphysis (SCFE) is a disorder that is more frequently found in boys than girls at a ratio of 3:1. Its peak frequency is reached in adolescence at the time of the most rapid growth phase (girls: 10–14 years; and boys: 11–15 years). In half of the children, this condition is bilateral and partially staggered over time.

In a Japanese multicentre study performed in 2002, Noguchi et al. [12] described a comparable incidence of this disease between genders (boys: 2.22/100,000; girls: 0.76/100,000) similar to that reported in the USA in 1970 by Kelsey et al. [13]. They attributed their finding to the similar increase in the number of obese children in Japan. The obesity index of the patients in this study was three times higher than that found in a comparative study carried out 30 years earlier [14].

Similar developments have been recently reported in Scotland, where data analysis showed an increase in the incidence of SCFE in children from 3.78/100,000 cases in 1981 to 9.66/100,000 cases in 2000 in addition to a lowering of the age in which this disease first manifests. In parallel, the National Obesity Prevention Programme in Scotland has documented a steady increase in the number of overweight school children over the past 20 years [15].

Pathogenesis

There is wide consensus that biomechanical as well as endocrinological factors play important roles in the aetiology of this disease. Often, there are conspicuous constitutional features in affected children and adolescents, such as truncal obesity accompanied by the underdevelopment of the genitals (dystrophia adiposogenitalis), and more rarely, somatomegaly.

Jingushi et al. [16] have discussed several theories on the aetiology of this disease and have provided pathogenetic models that draw upon extensive endocrinological, histomorphological and clinical data. Increased body weight in association with a growth spurt during puberty together with an increasingly oblique epiphyseal growth plate (retrotorsion of the femoral neck) are deemed essential risk factors.

Temporary changes in thyroid, growth and sex hormones during the period of rapid longitudinal growth lead to a loosening and expansion of the collagen network of the growth plate itself, with weakening of the perichondrial ring at the femoral neck. Resistance of the growth plate to shearing forces is thus diminished, and there is increased danger of epiphyseal dislocation. According to this hypothesis, obese children are particularly prone to epiphysiolysis during their pubertal growth phase. It is therefore even more important to make general practitioners, paediatricians and paediatric orthopaedic specialists/surgeons aware of this disease so that a slippage is diagnosed as early as possible, and adequate treatment is offered.

Clinical Findings and Diagnostics

Every episode of epiphysiolysis leads to more or less pronounced hip, thigh or knee complaints.

It is important to recognise that during the early stage of SCFE, clinical signs can be highly unspecific, and complaints are often underestimated over a longer period of time. If the slippage is advanced, there is a typical loss of internal rotation in the affected hip, which is described as 'Drehmann's sign' (fig. 4).

The diagnosis of SCFE is usually confirmed radiologically. It must be emphasised that with a dorsal slipping of the epiphyseal plate, a simple anteroposterior radiograph of the affected hip can frequently miss the incipient slippage. In the case of suspected femoral head slippage, two radiographic projections of the affected hip should be taken because the epiphyseal slippage is only discernible in the second projection (fig. 5).

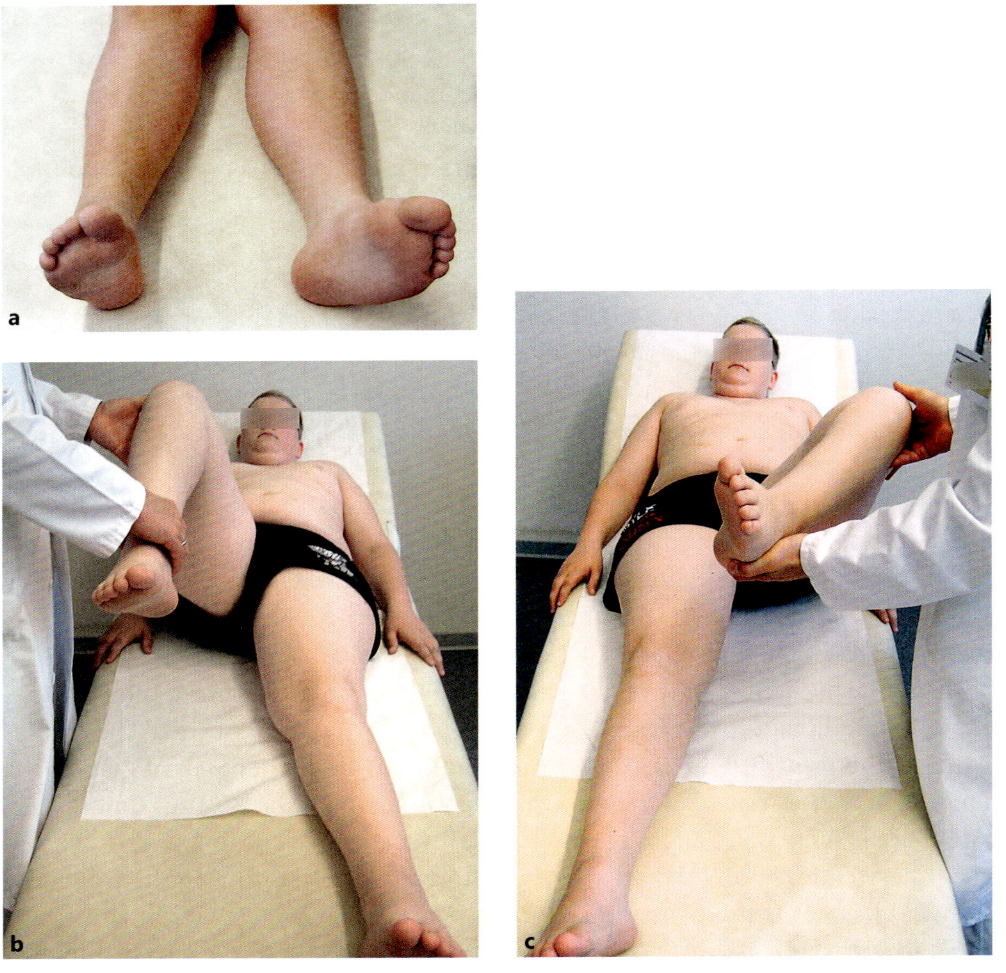

Fig. 4. Typical clinical findings of SCFE, including the spontaneous external rotation of the affected left leg (**a**) and the so-called Drehmann's sign of spontaneous abduction and external rotation of the affected left leg during passive or active bending of the hip (**b**, **c**).

Therapy

SCFE always requires immediate admission to the hospital for prompt surgical stabilisation of the epiphysis to prevent further slippage. In an unstable type of SCFE (i.e. children who are not able to walk anymore) or in cases in which the slippage has progressed to a considerable extent, even more invasive surgical techniques might be required.

Natural Course

Advanced stages of this disease carry a high risk of chondrolysis and lead to femoroacetabular impingement and joint incongruency. Therefore, these are important risk factors for the development of secondary OA.

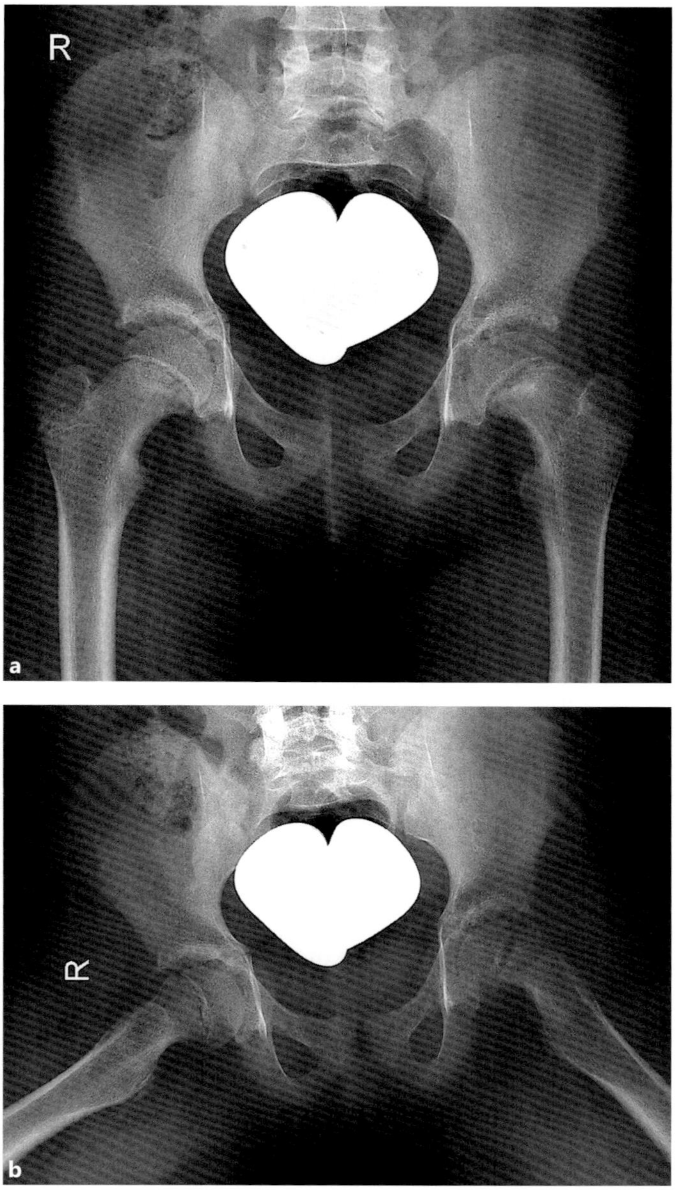

Fig. 5. Radiographic diagnosis of SCFE is always performed in 2 projections. In the pelvic overview radiograph (**a**), only a more severe loosening of the left epiphyseal plate is discernible. Only in the axial view (**b**), the advanced slippage of the left epiphyseal plate and the incipient dorsal slippage of the right epiphyseal plate are visible. The angle of slippage in each case can be measured.

Even mild epiphyseal slippage can lead to changes in the biomechanics and mobility of the hip joint. Over the long term, the resulting malformation at the junction of the femoral head-femoral neck (the so-called 'tilt' or 'pistol grip' deformity) represents a risk factor for cartilage degeneration. Extensive clinical and radiological investigations within the 'Ulm Osteoarthritis Study' showed, for instance, that 7.1% of study participants with advanced OA exhibited these typical radiological changes at the femoral head-femoral neck junction, which suggests that they had experienced a mild form of epiphyseal slippage within the context of SCFE [17].

Summary
SCFE is a multifactorial disease in which obesity plays an important aetiological role as a cofactor. This disease should be excluded with the help of radiographs in 2 projections (antero-posterior and lateral views) in cases of hip and knee complaints in children and adolescents before and during puberty that cannot be clearly classified by patient history and clinical presentation. Important sequelae of this disease (i.e. chondrolysis and secondary OA) must be prevented by its early diagnosis and appropriate therapy.

Obesity and Osteoarthritis

OA of large, load-bearing joints is one of the most frequent disorders of the musculoskeletal system and has high socio-medical significance [18]. In approximately 50% of affected individuals, it is possible to identify well-defined causes of this disease or associated risk factors. Childhood diseases that lead to severe deviations from anatomically correct joint morphology are designated as 'prearthroses'.

Data on clinical and radiological courses in patients with anatomically correct joint morphology but in whom the joints have been subjected to high mechanical loads due to long-term obesity are less clear. According to a report by 'Diabetes Australia', overweight is associated with a 1–2.45-fold increased risk of developing OA.

Epidemiological calculations show that in 2005, more than 225,000 Australians developed OA as a result of being overweight, which represents 14% of all Australian patients suffering from this disease [19]. Twenty years ago, several large studies [20, 21] pointed out a link between overweight and the development of knee OA. Felson et al. [21] investigated a cohort of female patients, reporting a decrease in the incidence of knee OA requiring treatment, which was achieved solely by weight reduction.

Within the Ulm Osteoarthritis Study, Stürmer et al. [22] also investigated associations between existing obesity and joint degeneration in men and women with advanced knee and hip OA necessitating joint replacement. In patients with advanced knee OA, such an association could be confirmed. This became even more evident by the finding of additional axis deviations in the related extremities. No relationship between body weight and bilateral hip OA, however, could be identified.

Influence of Overweight on Outcomes after Hip and Knee Replacements
In the presence of advanced OA that cannot be treated with conservative measures, joint replacement surgery is indicated. The main goal here is improvement of the quality of life in patients with severe joint complaints by enabling relief from pain and the improvement of joint function. In view of the increasingly improved prosthetic devices available with longer lives and increased durabilities that lead to higher patient satisfaction and reduced cost [23], there has been an increase worldwide in the total number of hip and knee replacements over the past few years.

The possible influence of obesity on patient outcome after joint replacement remains controversial. In an international multicentre cross-sectional study carried out within the framework of the EUROHIP, researchers found a lack of consensus between physicians in different specialties on the influence of overweight on hip replacement outcome. Thus, referring physicians were less likely to associate obesity with a favourable outcome after hip replacement than orthopaedic surgeons [24]. Many authors argue that overweight and obese patients are likely to not only be exposed to higher rates of general (e.g. thromboembolism) and special (e.g. bleeding, infection, aseptic implant loosening, and periprosthetic fracture) complications but also to derive less benefit from hip replacement compared to patients of normal weight [25]. On the other hand, there is also evidence that obese patients do not have to expect a poorer long-term outcome after hip replacement compared with people of normal weight [26, 27]. Within the framework of the Dresden Hip Surgery Registry [unpublished data], our prospective follow-up study with a large patient collective has suggested that overweight (BMI 25–30) or obesity (BMI >30) has no unfavourable effects on joint function or quality of life over the short- and medium-term after prosthetic hip implant.

Summary
The significance of local biomechanical and systemic-metabolic factors in the development of hip OA in the obese population remains controversial. An association between increased BMI and the development of knee OA, however, has been well established. It is unclear whether obese patients derive less benefit from total joint replacement than patients of normal weight based on the currently available literature.

Back Pain

Lumbar segments of the spine are most frequently affected by pain, which is mostly the consequence of the dysfunction or degeneration of the intervertebral discs or the small spinal joints with successive changes in the tones of the muscles and ligaments involved. During advanced stages of degeneration, protruding parts of intervertebral discs and segmental instability can lead to the compression of nerve roots with subsequent neurological symptoms (specific back pain). Inflammatory changes (i.e. spondylodiscitis) or tumours can also lead to back pain and must be excluded.

Whereas in adults and older people, overweight and obesity have been identified as important risk factors for the degeneration of intervertebral discs and development of back pain [28, 29], there are few studies investigating the association between spinal pain and truncal obesity in children and adolescents. Pain as a rule might be considered an early symptom of imminent degenerative changes. In this sense, risk factors

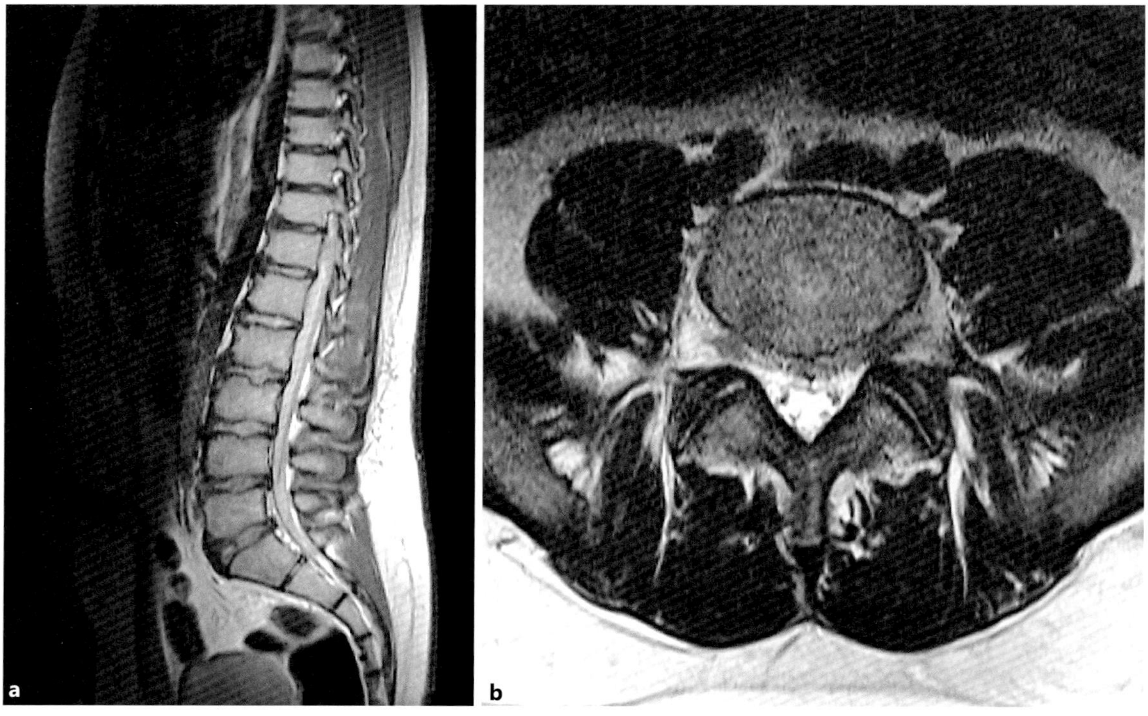

Fig. 6. a, b Atypical polysegmental lumbar changes seen in MRI associated with lumbar spinal stenosis in an overweight 14-year-old adolescent male (BMI 30.4) admitted to the hospital with acute pain and neurological deficits.

for intervertebral degeneration identified in adults must also be taken into consideration in children and adolescents with spinal complaints, and an appropriate treatment should be instituted. In a recent field study of 135 obese children and adolescents who underwent obesity counselling as part of their paediatric treatment, Stovitz et al. [30] reported that the majority of these children (61%) mentioned having pain once a month in at least one joint. In this population, the prevalence of back complaints was the highest (39%), with knee problems reported in 24%, ankle complaints in 15% and foot problems in 26% of the patients. Similar data have also been reported by Taylor et al. [31] and Bell et al. [32].

Early spinal changes atypical for this young age group, including neurological deficits, could also be observed in isolated adolescents with severe overweight in our patient collective (fig. 6).

Summary

Accumulating data on back pain in obese children and adolescents suggest an association between childhood obesity and the development of degenerative changes in the axial skeleton at a young age. In adult patients, the coincidence between degenerative changes in the spinal column and overweight is an established fact.

Conclusion

With the improvement of living standards and increasingly easy availability of food, there has been a parallel increase in the number of overweight people in developed countries over the course of many years. This fact has led not only to an increase in cardiovascular and metabolic diseases but also to an increased incidence of musculoskeletal complaints.

Inactivity resulting from such discomfort in many of those affected helps to maintain a vicious cycle that must be broken through early education and awareness for the establishment of alternative behaviours. In particular, there is sound scientific evidence linking degenerative (osteoarthritic) changes in the lumbar spine segments and the knee with overweight and obesity.

The frequency of diabetic foot problems increases with the duration of poorly managed diabetes mellitus. Diabetic foot syndrome is often underestimated and needs interdisciplinary care. Properly managed metabolic changes in diabetes, counselling and training, the correct treatment of wounds and orthopaedic diabetes footwear can often help to prevent complications.

Unfortunately, overweight and obesity and their consequences are observed not only in adults but also increasingly in children and adolescents. In particular, in the growing skeleton, overweight and obesity are associated with severe structural disturbances of the growth plates as well as secondary form and axis deviations in the load-bearing lower extremities. These axis deviations not only represent cosmetic and functional problems in the affected children and adolescents but also potentiate the subsequent risk of degenerative joint disorder (OA). Professional groups who are entrusted with the care of overweight children and adolescents should be aware of the frequent occurrence of disorders of the skeletal system within the context of specific developmental phases and should respond with particular sensitivity to early symptoms.

References

1 Horn MR: Orthopädische Komorbidität bei Kindern und Jugendlichen mit Adipositas unter besonderer Berücksichtigung der Epiphysiolysis capitis femoris; thesis, Universität Ulm, Ulm, 2002.

2 Riddiford-Harland DL, Steel JR, Storlien LH: Does obesity influence foot structure in prepubescent children? Int J Obes Relat Metab Disord 2000;24:541–544.

3 Dowling AM, Steel JR, Baur LA: Does obesity influence foot structure and plantar pressure patterns in prepubescent children. Int J Obes Relat Metab Disord 2001;25:845–852.

4 Dowling AM, Steel JR, Baur LA: What are the effects of obesity in children on plantar pressure distribution? Int J Obes 2004;28:1514–1519.

5 Bruckner L, Rosler P: Orthopaedic findings of the foot as related to age and body weight among women. ZFA 1981;36:29–35.

6 Mertz DP: [Hallux rigidus arthrosis and gout]. Fortschr Med 1982;100:446–448.

7 Hefti F: Achsenfehler an den unteren Extremitäten. Orthopäde 2000;29:814–820.

8 Blount WP: Tibia vara: osteochondrosis deformans tibiae. J Bone Joint Surg 1937;19A:1–8.

9 Davids JR, Huskamp M, Bagley AM: A dynamic biomechanical analysis of the etiology of adolescent tibia vara. J Pediatr Orthop 1996;16:461–468.
10 de Sá Pinto AL, de Barros Holanda PM, Radu AS, Villares SM, Lima FR: Musculoskeletal findings in obese children. J Peadiatr Child Health 2006;42:341–344.
11 White GR, Mencio GA: Genu valgum in children: diagnostic and therapeutic alternatives. J Am Acad Orthop Surg 1995;3:275–283.
12 Noguchi Y, Sakamaki T, Multicenter Study Committee of the Japanese Pediatric Orthopaedic Association: Epidemiology and demographic of slipped capital femoral epiphysis in Japan: a multi-center study by the Japanese Pediatric Orthopaedic Association. J Orthop Sci 2002;7:610–617.
13 Kelsey JL, Keggi KJ, Southwick WO: The incidence and distribution of slipped femoral epiphysis in Connecticut and Southwestern United States. J Bone Joint Surg 1970;52A:1203–1216.
14 Ninomiya S, Nagasaka Y, Tagawa H: Slipped capital femoral epiphysis: a study of 68 cases in the eastern half area of Japan. Clin Orthop 1976;119:172–176.
15 Murray AW, Wilson NIL: Changing incidence of slipped capital femoral epiphysis. A relationship with obesity? J Bone Joint Surg (Br) 2008;90-B:92–94.
16 Jingushi S, Suenaga E: Slipped capital femoral epiphysis: etiology and treatment. J Orthop Sci 2004;9: 214–219.
17 Günther KP, Stürmer T, Sauerland S, Zeissig I, Sun Y, Kessler S, Scharf HP, Brenner H, Puhl W: Prevalence of generalized osteoarthritis in patients with advanced hip and knee OA: the Ulm osteoarthritis study. Ann Rheum Dis 1998;57:717–723.
18 Günther KP, Merx H: Epidemiologie und sozialmedizinische bedeutung der arthrose; in Zacher J (ed): Herausforderung Arthrose. Berlin, Berufsverband der Fachärzte für Orthopädie, 2006.
19 Access Economics: The Economic Costs of Obesity. Canberra, Access-Economics, 2006.
20 Davis MA, Ettinger WH, Neuhaus JM: Obesity and osteoarthritis of the knee: evidence from the national health and nutrition examination survey (NHANES I). Semin Arthritis Rheum 1990;20:34–41.
21 Felson DT, Zhang Y, Anthony JM, Naimark A, Anderson JJ: Weight loss reduces the risk for symptomatic knee osteoarthritis in women. Ann Intern Med 1992;116:535–539.
22 Stürmer T, Günther KP, Brenner H: Obesity, overweight and patterns of osteoarthritis: the Ulm osteoarthritis study. J Clin Epidemiol 2000;53:307–313.
23 Katz JN: Preferences, quality, and the (under)utilization of total joint arthroplasty. Med Care 2001;39: 203–205.
24 Stürmer T, Dreinhofer K, Grober-Gratz D, Brenner H, Dieppe P, Puhl W, Günther KP: Differences in the views of orthopaedic surgeons and referring practitioners on the determinants of outcome after total hip replacement. J Bone Joint Surg Br 2005;87:1416–1419.
25 Namba RS, Paxton L, Fithian DC, Stone ML: Obesity and perioperative morbidity in total hip and total knee arthroplasty patients. J Arthroplasty 2005; 20(7 suppl 3):46–50.
26 Andrew JG, Palan J, Kurup HV, Gibson P, Murray DW, Beard DJ: Obesity in total hip replacement. J Bone Joint Surg Br 2008;90:424–429.
27 McLaughlin JR, Lee KR: The outcome of total hip replacement in obese and non-obese patients at 10- to 18-years. J Bone Joint Surg Br 2006;88:1286–1292.
28 Hangai M, Kaneoka K, Kuno S, Hinotsu S, Sakane M, Mamizuka N, Sakane M, Ochiai N: Factors associated with lumbar intervertebral disc degeneration in the elderly. Spine J 2008;8:732–740.
29 Shiri R, Solovieva S, Husgafvel-Pursiainen K, Taimela S, Saarikoski LA, Huupponen R, Viikari J, Raitakari OT, Viikari-Juntura E: The association between obesity and the prevalence of low back pain in young adults: the Cardiovascular Risk in Young Finns Study. Am J Epidemiol 2008;167:1110–1119.
30 Stovitz SD, Pardee PE, Vazquez G, Duval S, Schwimmer JB: Musculoskeletal pain in obese children and adolescents. Acta Paediatr 2008;97:489–493.
31 Taylor ED, Theim KR, Mirch MC, Ghorbani S, Tanofsky-Kraff M, Adler-Wailes DC, Brady S, Reynolds JC, Calis KA, Yanovski JA: Orthopedic complications of overweight in children and adolescents. Pediatrics 2006;117:2167–2174.
32 Bell LM, Byrne S, Thompson A, Ratnam N, Blair E, Bulsara M, Jones TW, Davis EA: Increasing body mass index z-score is continuously associated with complications of overweight in children, even in the healthy weight range. J Clin Endocrinol Metab 2007; 92:517–522.

Falk Thielemann, MD
University Centre of Orthopaedics and Traumatology
University Hospital Carl Gustav Carus at Technical University Dresden
Fetscherstrasse 74
DE–01307 Dresden (Germany)
E-Mail falk.thielemann@uniklinikum-dresden.de

Kiess W, Wabitsch M, Maffeis C, Sharma AM (eds): Metabolic Syndrome and Obesity in Childhood and Adolescence.
Pediatr Adolesc Med. Basel, Karger, 2015, vol 19, pp 99–109 (DOI: 10.1159/000368111)

Urogenital Complications: Renal Disease, Urolithiasis and Lower Urinary Tract Symptoms

Anita Morandi · Claudio Maffeis

Pediatric Diabetes, Clinical Nutrition and Obesity, Department of Life and Reproduction Science,
School of Medicine and Surgery, University of Verona, Verona, Italy

Abstract

The chapter contains a critical review of the current literature pertaining to the consequences of childhood and adolescent obesity/metabolic syndrome on the urogenital system, with a particular focus on microalbuminuria, renal disease, urolithiasis and lower urinary tract symptoms. The clinical implications of the current evidence with regard to the relationship between early obesity/metabolic syndrome and the above-mentioned conditions are discussed.

Renal Disease

Obesity and metabolic syndrome (MS) have been associated with renal damage in adults [1]. Obesity directly favors renal damage through several mechanisms [1] (fig. 1). The obesity-related activation of the renin-angiotensin-aldosterone system is one of the most extensively studied mechanisms explaining renal injury driven by obesity [1]. Adipocytes possess a renin-angiotensin system and produce angiotensin II, thus stimulating the production of aldosterone [1]. Moreover, adipose tissue also secretes angiotensin-independent mineralocorticoid-releasing factors [1]. Thus, obesity is associated with a state of hyperaldosteronism leading to plasma expansion, glomerular hyperfiltration and damage and proteinuria, which often occurs in parallel with a state of pre-hypertension [1]. Aldosterone has also been shown to have direct negative glomerular effects in animal models, independent of blood pressure and plasma expansion [1].

An obesity-associated decrease in adiponectin levels is another mechanism of renal damage because of the resultant reduced AMP-activated protein kinase in glomerular

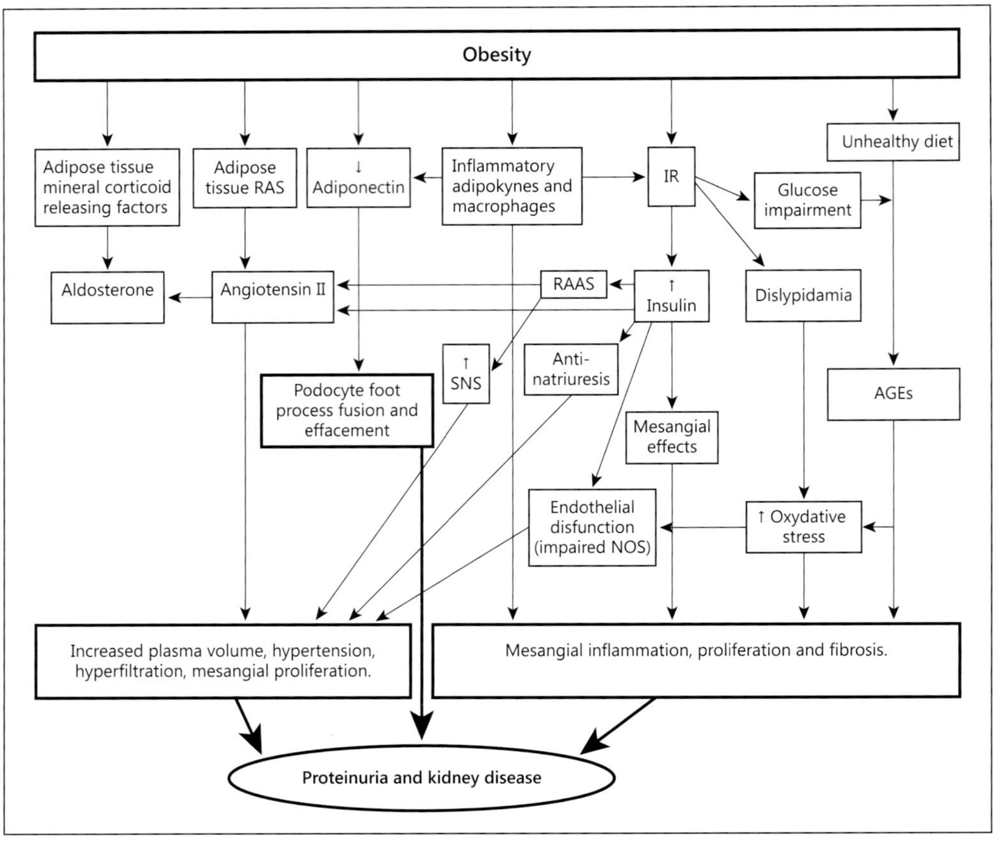

Fig. 1. Pathogenic pathways of renal damage associated with obesity and metabolic syndrome. RAS = renin-angiotensin system; RAAS = renin-angiotensin-aldosterone system; IR = insulin resistance; SNS = sympathetic nervous system; AGEs = advanced glycation end products; NOS = nitric oxide synthase.

podocytes with consequent podocyte foot process fusion and effacement [1]. Obesity is also associated with the overexpression of PA-1 and cytokines in both visceral tissue and glomeruli and with glomerular infiltration by proinflammatory macrophages, leading to renal inflammation, fibrosis and proteinuria [1].

Finally, an overload of dietary advanced glycation end products associated with obesity may be another cause of renal injury and proteinuria [1]. Apart from the direct effects of excessive adipose tissue on the kidney, obesity-related insulin resistance (IR)/hyperinsulinemia is a well-recognized cause of renal damage, even in the absence of diabetes [2]. In particular, insulin has an antinatriuretic effect, increasing sodium reabsorption without affecting the glomerular filtration rate or aldosterone levels [2]. Moreover, insulin affects the renin-angiotensin-aldosterone system, increasing its activity despite volume expansion [2]. It also increases the effects of angiotensin II on mesangial cells, thus favoring hypertension, increased intraglomerular pressure, proteinuria, and the production of renal cytokines and growth factors with consequent mesangial proliferation, fibrosis and apoptosis [2]. Insulin *per se* can promote mesangial proliferation and the production of extracellular matrix proteins [2]. Furthermore, it is thought to encourage renal damage by decreasing the production of endothelial nitric oxide, with consequent vasoconstriction and hypertension [2]. Finally, obesity and IR-related dyslipidemia are additional causes of renal damage because they promote inflammation and endothelial dysfunction [2].

Several longitudinal and cross-sectional studies on adults have shown significant associations between obesity and asymptomatic proteinuria, non-diabetic/non-hypertensive chronic kidney disease (CKD) and death from non-diabetic/non-hypertensive end-stage renal disease (ESRD) [1]. Moreover, the epidemic of severe obesity has been correlated with a ten-fold increase in the prevalence of a specific obesity-related CKD called obesity-related glomerulopathy (ORG), which is characterized by obesity-related glomerulomegaly alone or in association with focal segmental glomerulosclerosis (FSGS) and by nephrotic syndrome and chronic renal failure, with a lower rate of progression towards ESRD compared to idiopathic FSGS (3.6 vs. 42%, respectively) [1]. ORG is typical of severe obesity, and it can be estimated to affect 3–4% of severely obese adults in the United States (U.S.) according to epidemiological evidence on the overall prevalence of CKD, the percentage of CKD accounted for by ORG and the prevalence of severe obesity [1]. The relationships between obesity and pre-clinical renal damage, CKD and progression towards ESRD in children and adolescents have not been extensively investigated. The following paragraphs contain a critical review of current literature pertaining to the associations between obesity/MS and microalbuminuria (MA), CKD, and the progression of renal damage in children and adolescents.

Microalbuminuria

The association between MA and pediatric obesity/MS is complex. In 2008, the National Health and Nutrition Education Study (NHANES) [3] defined MA as an albumin-to-creatinine ratio (ACR) of 30–300 mg/g that was negatively associated with overweight/obesity in 2,515 adolescents with an overall prevalence of MA of 8.9%. In the NHANES [3], normal-weight adolescents had an 8.7% prevalence of MA, and it was 0.3% in overweight/obese adolescents. Consistently, a more recent study on 1,564 Argentinean children has reported that obese children are less likely than normal-weight children to present with an ACR of above the median, and a study on 365 Greek adolescents has reported an inverse correlation between the ACR and standardized body mass index (Z-BMI) [4, 5]. This body of evidence underscores the notion that childhood and adolescent obesity are not risk factors for MA at the community level and are even associated with lower prevalences of MA and lower ACRs. The reason for this unexpected association is unknown, but authors have generally argued that lean children and adolescents are more likely to have orthostatic and exercise-related proteinuria than their overweight counterparts [3–5].

On the other hand, several referral-based studies have consistently shown that among obese adolescent outpatients, those who have an insulin-resistant phenotype; for example, higher fasting or post-challenge insulin and/or glucose and/or more severe obesity, are at increased risk for MA [6–10]. Furthermore, the NHANES [3] reported that cardiovascular risk factors (impaired fasting glucose, IR, hypertension and smoking) were associated with MA among overweight and obese adolescents but not among normal-weight participants, suggesting that obesity-mediated IR is the key pathogenetic link between cardiovascular risk factors and MA among adolescents. The NHANES [3] has indicated that IR as defined as a homeostasis model assessment of IR (HOMA-IR) of ≥4 (15% of subjects) is the strongest risk factor for MA, with an unadjusted odds ratio (OR) of 19 [1.89–189]. In contrast, MS, lipid levels and blood pressure have not always been proven to be predictors of MA in obese children and adolescents [7, 9, 11]. Studies on diabetic youth have further reinforced the notion that IR is an important causative risk factor for MA. In particular, the SEARCH for Diabetes in Youth study [12] has reported that among 3,259 diabetic adolescents, those with type 1 diabetes have a 9.2% prevalence of MA, and those with type 2 diabetes have a 22.2% prevalence; in addition, the association between type 2 diabetes and MA is strongly attenuated by adjustments for obesity, hypertension and triglycerides. More recently, the same study has reported that the subsample of diabetic adolescents without diabetes autoantibodies and with IR has a greater ACR compared with all other groups, possibly because of the greater magnitude of IR observed in this group [13]. Thus, evidence in the current literature suggests that obesity-related IR and glucose dysregulation are consistent risk factors for MA in youth.

The evidence that obesity is a risk factor for IR-related MA or severe obesity-related MA has given rise to the question of whether obese children and adolescents should be screened for MA despite the overall lower prevalence of this condition among obese compared with normal-weight youth. The overall low prevalence (2–3%) of MA observed in multi-ethnic or mainly European referral-based cohorts of obese children and adolescents argues against the routine assessment of MA in asymptomatic obese patients [3, 7, 14]. Populations of non-European ancestry are known to have a higher prevalence of MA than European populations [15]. A referral-based study on 150 obese Egyptian children reported a 14.7% prevalence of MA, suggesting that the debate on the cost-effectiveness of routine MA assessment in obese pediatric patients could be more worthwhile for certain non-European populations [6]. Evidence supporting the assessment of MA in sub-groups of obese patients presenting with risk factors like IR, glucose dysregulation or very high BMI is also scarce. In fact, most studies of risk factors for MA do not contain any analysis of the association between MA and risk factors but simply report on the relationship between the ACR and metabolic risk factors or ACRs above the median and metabolic risk factors [4, 5, 7, 8, 10, 11]. Thus, these studies do not help to assess the accuracy of metabolic risk factors in discriminating obese patients with MA, and consequently, they do not help to evaluate the potential clinical values of these factors. Among the few studies analyzing the associations between metabolic/anthropometric risk factors and MA, the NHANES [3] has indicated that a HOMA-IR of ≥4 could be a very sensitive criterion to detect cases of MA in obese adolescents. In fact, the very strong association between a HOMA-IR of ≥4 and MA that has been reported by the NHANES (unadjusted OR = 19 [1.89–189]) [3] implies that almost all cases of MA are characterized by a HOMA-IR of ≥4. However, due to the very low prevalence of MA, almost all obese adolescents with this risk factor do not have this condition; therefore, the HOMA-IR, despite its sensitivity, would be a poor specific and predictive risk factor, or in other words, it would have a very low diagnostic yield if adopted for the detection of MA cases (approximately 1 case for every 20 tests). An HOMA-IR of ≥4.34 has been proven to be associated with MA in the above-mentioned referral-based Egyptian cohort, but despite the higher prevalence of MA in this cohort compared with the NHANES (14.7 vs. 0.3%), this criterion would not be a satisfactory screening tool for detecting patients likely to have MA because of its moderate strength of association in this sample (OR = 2.14 [1.15–5.53]), implying a low sensitivity for detecting the screened condition [6]. Another recent study on 408 obese children and adolescents with a 2.7% prevalence of MA failed to find any association between MA and the HOMA-IR, but the HOMA-IR cut-off used as a potential screening tool was 3.5, not 4 or 4.34 [14]. Importantly, not only were the three above-mentioned studies heterogeneous with regard to ethnicity, type of recruitment and the criteria adopted to define IR, but they also included a total of 42 patients with MA; therefore, they were underpowered to provide precise estimations of the predictive properties of IR as a risk factor for MA, as confirmed by the large confidence intervals of the ORs associated with IR [3, 6, 14]. This is significant because in a population with an approximately 15% prevalence of MA, such as that in the Egyptian study, an OR of 5.1 instead of 2.14 could make the difference between the clinical utility or nonutility of the HOMA-IR as a screening tool for selecting obese children to undergo urinalysis. Similar conclusions can be made for other metabolic or anthropometric risk factors taken into consideration by the cited studies. Finally, it must be pointed out that even if highly discriminative risk factors for MA exist, its assessment in obese children who test positive for such factors would not be justified because its exact prognostic value in obese children or adolescents has not yet been elucidated, and a specific therapy for isolated MA in obese youth does not yet exist.

Overall, it can be concluded that current evidence does not support the assessment of MA in all obese pediatric patients nor in sub-groups at higher risk. Especially for non-European populations, studies on large referral-based cohorts of obese children and adolescents are warranted to better define the potential utility of IR-related variables in selecting obese youth who should undergo a urinalysis to assess the extent of albuminuria. In parallel, longitudinal studies investigating the prognosis of early MA in obese patients and possibly clinical trials investigating therapeutic options are needed to justify the screening of MA in obese children.

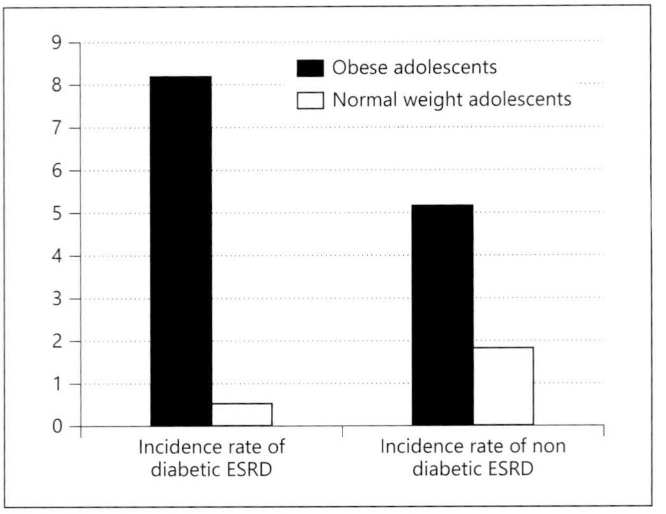

Fig. 2. Incidence rates per 100,000 person-years of diabetic and non-diabetic ESRDs in obese and normal-weight adolescents according to Vivante et al. [16].

Chronic Kidney Disease

A prospective study on approximately 1.2 million adolescents from Israel with an overall ESRD incidence of 2.87 cases per 100,000 person-years reported an incidence rate of 13.4 cases per 100,000 person-years in obese adolescents [16]. This incidence rate was accounted for by an 8.1 incidence rate of diabetic ESRD and a 5.1 incidence rate of non-diabetic ESRD (fig. 2). Even after adjustment for hypertension and other confounders, adolescent obesity was associated with nearly a 20-fold higher risk of diabetic ESRD and a 3.41-fold higher risk of non-diabetic ESRD [16]. This robust evidence, which is consistent with longitudinal data from adult populations, proves that adolescent obesity is not only associated with diabetic nephropathy but also with obesity-related CKD and/or with a higher rate of progression of all types of non-diabetic CKD [16]. Unfortunately, this study did not allow for the dissecting of the diverse causes of non-diabetic ESRD associated with adolescent obesity, although it emphasized a significantly higher rate of progression towards ESRD due to CKD in obese compared to normal-weight adolescents [16]. Moreover, all adolescents with baseline proteinuria were excluded; thus, this study did not help to determine the prognostic significance of asymptomatic proteinuria in obese adolescents [16]. Finally, it was not multi-ethnic [16]. The only other available prospective study on early life overweight and subsequent renal function, which assessed the relationship between early life overweight and CKD, was much less powerful than the above-mentioned study [17]. This longitudinal study was on a British cohort of 4,340 participants followed from 2 to 60–64 years of age, with an overall 1.7% prevalence of CKD defined as a cystatin-based estimated GFR (eGFRcys) of less than 60 ml/min/1.73 m^2. In this cohort, prepuberty and puberty onset long-standing obesity were associated with approximately twice the risk of developing eGFRcys-defined CKD at 60–64 years of age

[17]. This association was strongly attenuated after adjustments for the presence of diabetes and hypertension, but the authors acknowledged the probable lack of statistical power to detect any association between early obesity and later non-diabetic/non-hypertensive CKD [17]. Of note, the association between early obesity and CKD was not significant when the creatinine-based estimated GFR (eGFRcr) was adopted instead of the eGFRcys [17]. This may be partially because CKD was overestimated at the highest BMI levels by the eGFRcys compared to the eGFRcr, favoring the higher incidence of CKD in the class of individuals with long-standing obesity from childhood/adolescence to adult life because of misclassification. Thus, the association between early life obesity and later CKD highlighted by this study should be considered with caution [18]. Overall, the results of the above-mentioned longitudinal studies prove that adolescent obesity surely increases the risk of suffering from diabetic and non-diabetic ESRD, raises the risk of diabetic or hypertensive CKD and perhaps also increases the risk of suffering from any form of non-diabetic/non-hypertensive CKD in adulthood.

Cross-sectional studies that have assessed the association between the eGFR and BMI during childhood and adolescence have produced conflicting results. The most powerful study (the CREDIT study [19]) showed that among 3,622 5- to 18-year-old Turkish children, obese participants and those with hypercholesterolemia had a lower (not better specified) mean eGFRcr compared to normal weight participants but did not have different rates of eGFRcr <90 or <75 ml/min/1.73 m^2. In contrast, a small previous study on 166 healthy Greek children and adolescents has reported that obesity and MS are associated with a higher eGFRcr, suggesting that obesity and the related metabolic impairment may involve renal hyperfiltration as a possible first step towards renal damage [20]. A third study on 113 obese Iranian adolescents has reported that the presence of MS is a risk factor for a lower eGFRcr [21]. Interestingly, none of these studies were based on direct measurements of GFR but on creatinine-based estimates of the GFR. The impact of obesity and body composition on the accuracy of the eGFRcr in children and adolescents has not yet been elucidated, and consequently, methods to adjust the eGFRcr for these variables are not yet available. However, there is evidence that creatinine-based methods may overestimate the GFR in obese individuals because of the increased tubular secretion of creatinine at the highest BMI levels [22]. On the other hand, the use of body surface in the eGFRcr formula may not be sufficient to account for the higher absolute lean mass and subsequent higher creatinine production in obese children and adolescents, implying an underestimation of the GFR in obese youth with a good percentage of fat-free mass. Thus, the above-mentioned body of evidence on the cross-sectional association between obesity/MS and GFR in childhood/adolescence could be biased by a latent systematic over- or under-estimation of the GFR according to anthropometric variables. In the future, large studies with direct measurements of or BMI/fatness-adjusted estimates of the GFR in multi-ethnic cohorts of children and adolescents will be necessary to unravel the role of BMI/MS on renal function during childhood and adolescence. At the moment, based on the results of the CREDIT study, it may be concluded that the GFR most likely does not differ or differs very modestly between obese and non-obese children and adolescents [19].

With regard to the current literature pertaining to ORG during childhood and adolescence, twelve years ago, a case report was published describing seven severely obese African American adolescents affected by nephrotic proteinuria and renal damage, including glomerular hypertrophy, FSGS, increased mesangial matrix and cellularity, the relative preservation of foot process morphology and the absence of evidence of inflammatory or immune-mediated pathogenesis [23]. In 2009, a multi-ethnic cohort study of 40 children and adolescents with non-diabetic kidney disease and proteinuria and with available renal biopsies has reported that the FSGS of obese patients is typically associated with glomerulomegaly in contrast with that of non-obese patients and is characterized by a slower progression towards ESRD, unless the obesity is associated with pre-term birth [24]. Evidence of the exact prevalence and prognosis of ORG in severely obese children and adolescents is lacking.

Urolithiasis

Adult obesity is positively associated with the prevalence and incidence of kidney stones, and the strongest association is with uric acid stones, although the extent to which obesity influences each type of stone is still unknown [1]. Recently, a large hospital-based case-control study on 9,843 pediatric cases of urolithiasis and 39,047 age- and hospital-matched controls has reported that this condition is associated with higher odds of obesity (OR = 1.30 [1.12–1.51]), suggesting that obesity is a risk factor for urolithiasis among pediatric patients at freestanding children's hospitals [25]. In contrast, a study comparing the prevalence of obesity among 222 pediatric patients with urolithiasis to that of the general pediatric population and two studies comparing the prevalence of obesity among 297 pediatric patients with urolithiasis to that among 674 healthy controls did not find any associations between obesity and urolithiasis [26–28]. Thus, obesity could be a risk factor for kidney stones among hospital-recruited children but not in the general pediatric population. Larger population-based studies are needed to clarify this point.

Two studies comparing 293 obese children to 331 normal-weight children have reported that obesity is associated with urinary risk factors for stone formation, such as lower pH, higher oxalate and lower citrate concentrations [29, 30]. This suggests that during childhood, urinary risk factors for kidney stone formation are associated with obesity. A recent study has reported that among 46 obese adolescents, IR and the number of risk factors for MS are associated with lower urinary pH and a higher relative saturation ratio of calcium oxalate, which are two important risk factors for kidney stone formation [31]. Thus, IR and MS may trigger the formation of kidney stones among obese adolescents.

Lower Urinary Tract Symptoms

Childhood obesity is associated with enuresis [32, 33]. According to a recent study on 281 children and adolescents, obese children are approximately three times more prone to suffer from enuresis than normal-weight children (30 vs. 8.8%) [32]. Moreover, in this study, obesity was shown to explain the association between enuresis and attention- deficit/hyperactivity disorder [32]. Unhealthy diets that overwhelm functional bladder capacity, psychological distress and parental indulgence have been proposed as potential explanations for obesity-associated enuresis [32]. According to previous data, childhood obesity is associated not only with enuresis but also with a higher rate of treatment failure among enuretic children and a lower voiding diary completion [33]. Authors agree that enuresis should be clarified during the primary workup of every obese child and adolescent [32, 33].

Similar to what is observed in obese adult women, obesity is associated with stress urinary incontinence (SUI) in obese adolescents [34, 35]. The exact prevalence of this complication among obese girls is not known but may be approximately 10% in contrast to its virtual absence among normal-weight healthy girls [34]. Severe adolescent female SUI, which is estimated to be rare, has also been reported as a comorbidity of obesity in adolescent girls [35]. It is characterized by the leakage of large amounts of urine at least once weekly, and its severity may require surgical treatment because of the ineffectiveness of antimuscarinic medications and physiotherapy [35]. The mechanism behind the association of obesity with SUI is unknown [1]. However, it is hypothesized that obesity increases abdominal pressure, which raises bladder pressure and urethral mobility, leading to SUI [1]. The increase in intravesical pressure created by obesity may reduce the continence gradient between the bladder and urethra, leading to higher static pressure within the bladder, thus reducing the magnitude of increase in intra-abdominal pressure necessary to force urine through the urethra [1].

Overall Summary

Obesity and MS favor renal damage in several ways. While common obesity does not seem to increase the risk of MA among children and adolescents, severely obese adolescents with IR could develop this condition. The prognosis of MA in obese adolescents is not known, and there is currently no strategy to accurately select obese children and adolescents at higher risk of MA and to test them for this condition. Longstanding obesity of pre-pubertal or pubertal onset is associated with increased risks of diabetic and non-diabetic ESRD, but it is not clear whether early obesity is associated with a higher prevalence of non-diabetic CKD during adulthood. Only a few cases of ORG have been reported in severely obese adolescents. Data on the GFR-obesity relationship during childhood and adolescence are based on estimated measurements that are likely to be influenced by BMI and are not conclusive; thus, they do not allow for the routine assessment of renal function among obese children and adolescents. Apart from hospital-based cohorts, obesity does not seem to increase the prevalence of kidney stones among children and adolescents, even when obesity and MS are associated with increased urinary risk factors for stone formation. Obesity is associated with pediatric enuresis and female stress urinary incontinence, which should be assessed during the primary workup of obese children and adolescents.

References

1 Morandi A, Maffeis C: Urogenital complications of obesity. Best Pract Res Clin Endocrinol Metab 2013; 27:209–218.

2 Savino A, Pelliccia P, Chiarelli F, et al: Obesity-related renal injury in childhood. Horm Res Paediatr 2010;73:303–311.

3 Nguyen S, McCulloch C, Brakeman P, et al: Being overweight modifies the association between cardiovascular risk factors and microalbuminuria in adolescents. Pediatr 2008;121:37–45.

4 Hirschler V, Molinari C, Maccallini G, et al: Is albuminuria associated with obesity in school children? Ped Diab 2010;11:322–330.

5 Mazaraki A, Tsioufis C, Dimitriadis K, et al: Adherence to the Mediterranean diet and albuminuria levels in Greek adolescents: data from the Leontio Lyceum ALbuminuria (3L study). Eur J Clin Nutr 2011; 65:219–225.

6 Sanad M, Gharib A: Evaluation of microalbuminuria in obese children and its relation to metabolic syndrome. Pediatr Nephrol 2011;26:2193–2199.

7 Lurbe E, Torro MI, Alvarez J, et al: Prevalence and factors related to urinary albumin excretion in obese youths. J Hypertens 2013;31:2230–2236.

8 Verhulst SL, van Hoeck K, Schrauwen N, et al: Sleep-disordered breathing and proteinuria in overweight and obese children and adolescents. Horm Res 2008; 70:224–229.

9 Burgert TS, Dziura J, Yeckel C, et al: Microalbuminuria in pediatric obesity: prevalence and relation to other cardiovascular risk factors. Int J Obes (Lond) 2006;30:273–280.

10 Savino A, Pelliccia P, Giannini C, et al: Implications for kidney disease in obese children and adolescents. Pediatr Nephrol 2011;26:749–758.

11 Di Bonito P, Moio N, Scilla C, et al: Preclinical manifestations of organ damage associated with the metabolic syndrome and its factors in outpatient children. Atherosclerosis 2010;213:611–615.

12 Maahs DM, Snively BM, Bell RA, et al: Higher prevalence of elevated albumin excretion in youth with type 2 than type 1 diabetes: the SEARCH for Diabetes in Youth study. Diabetes Care 2007;30:2593–2598.

13 Mottl AK, Lauer A, Dabelea D, et al: Albuminuria according to status of autoimmunity and insulin sensitivity among youth with type 1 and type 2 diabetes. Diabetes Care 2013;36:3633–3638.

14 Radhakishun NNE, van Vliet M, von Rosenstiel IA, et al: Limited value of routine microalbuminuria assessment in multi-ethnic obese children. Pediatr Nephrol 2013;28:1145–1149.

15 Ogunniyi MO, Croft JB, Greenlund KJ, et al: Racial/ethnic differences in microalbuminuria among adults with prehypertension and hypertension: National Health and Nutrition Examination Survey (NHANES), 1999–2006. Am J Hypertens 2010;23: 859–864.

16 Vivante A, Golan E, Tzur D, et al: Body mass index in 1.2 million adolescents and risk for end-stage renal disease. Arch Intern Med 2012;172:1644–1650.

17 Silverwood RJ, Pierce M, Hardy R, et al: Scientific and data collection teams: early-life overweight trajectory and CKD in the 1946 British birth cohort study. Am J Kidney Dis 2013;62:276–284.

18 Vupputuri S, Fox CS, Coresh J, et al: Differential estimation of CKD using creatinine- versus cystatin C-based estimating equations by category of body mass index. Am J Kidney Dis 2009;53:993–1001.

19 Soylemezoglu O, Duzova A, Yalçinkaya F, et al: Chronic renal disease in children aged 5–18 years: a population-based survey in Turkey, the CREDIT-C study. Nephrol Dial Transplant 2012;27(Suppl 3): iii146–iii151.

20 Koulouridis E, Georgalidis K, Kostimpa I, et al: Metabolic syndrome risk factors and estimated glomerular filtration rate among children and adolescents. Pediatr Nephrol 2010;25:491–498.

21 Kelishadi R, Gheissari A, Bazookar N, et al: Kidney function in obese adolescents with or without metabolic syndrome in a nationally-representative sample of pediatric population: first report from the Middle East and North Africa: the CASPIAN-III Study: a Case-Control Study. J Res Med Sci 2013;18: 178–183.

22 Sinkeler SJ, Visser FW, Krikken JA, et al: Higher body mass index is associated with higher fractional creatinine excretion in healthy subjects. Nephrol Dial Transplant 2011;26:3181–3188.
23 Adelman RD, Restaino IG, Alon US, et al: Proteinuria and focal segmental glomerulosclerosis in severely obese adolescents. J Pediatr 2001;138:481–485.
24 Abitbol CL, Chandar J, Rodríguez MM, et al: Obesity and preterm birth: additive risks in the progression of kidney disease in children. Pediatr Nephrol 2009;24:1363–1370.
25 Kokorowski PJ, Routh JC, Hubert KC, et al: Association of urolithiasis with systemic conditions among pediatric patients at children's hospitals. J Urol 2012; 188(4 Suppl):1618–1622.
26 Penido MG, Srivastava T, Alon US: Pediatric primary urolithiasis: 12-year experience at a Midwestern Children's Hospital. J Urol 2013;189:1493–1497.
27 Selimoğlu MA, Menekşe E, Tabel Y: Is urolithiasis in children associated with obesity or malnutrition? J Ren Nutr 2013;23:119–122.
28 Kim SS, Luan X, Canning DA, et al: Association between body mass index and urolithiasis in children. J Urol 2011;186(4 Suppl):1734–1739.
29 Borysewicz-Sańczyk H, Porowski T, Hryniewicz A, et al: Urolithiasis risk factors in obese and overweight children. Pediatr Endocrinol. Diabetes Metab 2012;18:53–57.
30 Sarica K, Eryildirim B, Yencilek F, et al: Role of overweight status on stone-forming risk factors in children: a prospective study. Urology 2009;73:1003–1007.
31 Tiwari R, Campfield T, Wittcopp C, et al: Metabolic syndrome in obese adolescents is associated with risk for nephrolithiasis. J Pediatr 2012;160:615–620.
32 Weintraub Y, Singer S, Alexander D, et al: Enuresis – an unattended comorbidity of childhood obesity. Int J Obes (Lond) 2013;37:75–78.
33 Guven A, Giramonti K, Kogan BA: The effect of obesity on treatment efficacy in children with nocturnal enuresis and voiding dysfunction. J Urol 2007;178: 1458–1462.
34 Schwartz B, Wyman JF, Thomas W, et al: Urinary incontinence in obese adolescent girls. J Pediatr Urol 2009;5:445–450.
35 Haylen BT, Avery D, Chiu TL: Severe adolescent female stress urinary incontinence (SAFSUI): case report and literature review. Int Urogynecol J 2013;25: 393–396.

Anita Morandi, MD, PhD
Pediatric Diabetes, Clinical Nutrition and Obesity
Department of Life and Reproduction Science
School of Medicine and Surgery, University of Verona
4, Via Bengasi, IT–37134 Verona (Italy)
E-Mail anita.morandi@voila.fr

Kiess W, Wabitsch M, Maffeis C, Sharma AM (eds): Metabolic Syndrome and Obesity in Childhood and Adolescence.
Pediatr Adolesc Med. Basel, Karger, 2015, vol 19, pp 110–125 (DOI: 10.1159/000368112)

Influences of Childhood Obesity on Pubertal Development

Isabel V. Wagner[a, b] · Matthew Sabin[c] · Wieland Kiess[a]

[a]Department of Women and Child Health, Hospital for Children and Adolescents, University of Leipzig, Leipzig, and [b]IFB AdiposityDiseases, Medical Faculty, University of Leipzig, Leipzig, Germany; [c]Murdoch Childrens Research Institute and University of Melbourne, Parkville, Vic., Australia

Abstract

The process of pubertal development is only partly understood but is thought to be influenced by many partially unknown factors. During the 20th century, there was a secular trend towards earlier pubertal development. Due to the rising epidemic of childhood obesity, the relationship between body composition in childhood and the tempo and timing of puberty needs to be better understood. Studies have shown that there is a clear relation between reaching a critical body weight and pubertal onset and course. Moreover, a rapid and early weight gain during infancy, and even during foetal life, is associated with an earlier onset of menarche, an earlier pubertal growth spurt, an earlier thelarche in girls, an earlier pubarche in both sexes and an earlier increase in testicular volume in boys. Furthermore, there is a clear correlation between increasing body mass index and earlier pubertal development in girls. In boys, controversial data exist. The majority of studies propose that puberty and voice break occur earlier in obese boys when compared with normal-weight peers, but interestingly, a few studies show the opposite finding. The earlier onset of puberty that occurs in obese individuals could be mediated by factors that are directly linked to adipose tissue or could be an indirect effect of genetic and/or environmental factors. This review presents the current evidence on this topic, highlighting inconsistencies and opportunities for future research.

Introduction

Overweight and obesity are defined by the World Health Organization as abnormal or excessive fat accumulation that may impair health. In 2011, more than 40 million children under the age of five were overweight. Overweight in childhood is defined as a body mass index (BMI) above the 85th percentile and lower than the 95th percentile, whereas obesity is defined as a BMI above the 95th percentile. Puberty is the process of physical change by which a child's body matures into an adult body that is capable of sexual reproduction to enable fertilisation. Puberty is initiated by hormonal signals from the brain to the gonads: the ovaries in a girl, and the testes in a boy. On average, girls begin puberty at ages 9–11, and boys begin puberty at ages 10–12; girls usually complete puberty by ages 15–17, while boys usually complete puberty by ages 16–17.

To induce pubertal development, children need to have reached a certain body weight or at least a particular amount of fat [1–3]. Being underweight due to a condition such as anorexia nervosa, chronic illness or malnutrition can lead to delayed puberty and later subfertility. From the 20th century onwards, there has been a downward trend towards an earlier age at menarche that was thought to be due to improvements in nutrition and overall quality of life. This trend has now stabilised in many countries [4–7], but some countries, including the USA [8], Greece [9], and Jamaica [10], still report an advanced pubertal onset in their paediatric populations.

The increasing prevalence of obesity during childhood and adolescence is one of the major health problems in developed countries across Europe and in Canada and the USA, and this is a well-known statistic. However, obesity is also emerging as a significant problem in developing countries, where obesity and under-nutrition often co-exist [11]. The development of early comorbidities, including insulin resistance, dyslipidaemia, hypertension and other cardiovascular risk factors are often seen in overweight and obese youth, and metabolic syndrome is a diagnosis that is now often made on a regular basis in paediatric centres. Another complication, which is the major focus of this chapter, is the induction of earlier pubertal development in obese children [12–15]. Early puberty can lead to an imbalance in sexual and psychosocial maturation that can induce future health problems [16, 17]. Many previous studies have indicated a reasonably strong relationship between over-nutrition and the timing of puberty, giving rise to the critical mass theory [18]. This theory suggests that there is a critical fat mass (~17% body weight) required for menarche and a higher fat mass (22% body weight) needed to maintain reproductive capacity.

Given this relationship and the increasing prevalence of overweight and obese youths across the world, should we therefore expect a corresponding secular change in the timing of puberty [18]? At the moment, the data on this topic are controversial, and there is currently not enough evidence showing a direct association between global changes in obesity rates and early sexual maturation across the world. This article will therefore highlight and discuss the data that are available on this important but controversial topic. Due to the inconsistencies of the published data, it is necessary that we begin to plan new and interdisciplinary studies, ideally involving large numbers of youth who are followed over long periods of time, to better understand the trends in pubertal development. These types of studies also need to be linked to in vitro and in vivo investigations of the molecular mechanisms that govern puberty induction to find the missing links between adipose tissue and pubertal development [17, 19, 20].

Obesity

Childhood obesity is now a frequently seen condition, and its prevalence has only recently stabilised in many countries, including Germany [21]. However, the prevalence of childhood obesity is still much too high and even continues to rise in several countries around the world. Weight gain is the result of many different and diverse factors, such as exposure to an obesogenic environment and genetic traits that have evolved over time to facilitate fat storage [15, 22–25]. Children with lifestyle-induced obesity are often tall during childhood but have a normal final height, and this is often due to earlier (but still within the normal range) timing of pubertal development and hence earlier closure of the growth plates. Children who suffer from obesity due to specific genetic and/or hormonal conditions tend to be shorter than their predicted final height. These findings show that there are likely factors that affect both puberty and body composition [26–31].

Around 40–70% of the inter-individual differences in body weight can be explained by genetic variation – particularly in young children. Many different genes have been identified that impact body weight [32]. During evolution, different gene variants that guaranteed survival, even in times of malnutrition and starvation, have been selected. However, those conditions do not exist in our modern and obesogenic environment, and therefore, the selection of genes that promote overweight and obesity have become detrimental, leading to the development of weight-related metabolic complications [22, 33–35].

Furthermore, sociocultural surroundings can influence the development of obesity. For example, Christakis and Fowler have shown that an increase in body weight in one person can affect the body weight of friends, siblings, relatives and neighbours. Network phenomena, therefore, also seem to be relevant to the biological and behavioural traits of obesity, and obesity appears to spread through social ties [23, 36].

Pubertal Development

Puberty usually follows a typical pattern of development in both sexes. In girls, puberty usually starts at 9–14 years of age with breast development followed by pubic hair growth. In boys, true puberty starts at 10–15 years of age with an increase in testicular volume followed by pubic hair and enlargement of the penis. Pubertal development starts with activation of the hypothalamic-pituitary-gonadal axis. Changes in the production of the hypothalamic gonadotropin-releasing hormone (GnRH), the gonadotropins luteinising hormone (LH) and follicle-stimulating hormone and the sex steroids estradiol and testosterone lead to the manifestation of the first clinical signs of puberty. Pubic hair can develop independently from the activation of the hypothalamic-pituitary-gonadal axis (termed pubarche), for example, due to androgen production in the adrenal glands [22]; this phase is termed adrenarche and does not represent true puberty. Clinically, pubertal status can be classified with the help of the Tanner stages (B1–5 for breast development, P1–6 for pubic hair development, and G1–5 for male genitalia development). Unfortunately, this method is biased by the subjective evaluation of the examination and can therefore lead to problems in clinical studies. However, one has to take into consideration that, in some cases, obese girls may have suffered from pseudo- or lipogynaecomastia instead of real thelarche. All pubertal changes usually occur over a period of 4–5 years. The beginning, duration and maturation of puberty are a result of a complex interplay between the central nervous system, endocrine glands and adipose tissue [37, 38]. Interestingly, the timing of puberty is often markedly different between different ethnicities [21], and there is also a large variation in the timing of puberty, which can vary by up to 4 years, in any given population.

An increase of the hypothalamic secretion of GnRH is an essential step for activating the pituitary-gonadal axis at the start of pubertal development. A short phase of GnRH system activation occurs during foetal development and during the neonatal period; however, reactivation in later childhood is thought to be critical for the induction of puberty, and sudden changes in GnRH secretion are the inductor, timer and supporter of pubertal maturation. The activation of the system underlies large inter-individual variations that reflect the complexity of puberty and indicate that puberty is not simply a function of chronological age. The mechanisms that impact the GnRH secretory network convey information about metabolic fuels, energy stores and somatic development. The primary activation of GnRH during the foetal and neonatal periods and the intensity of this initial activation might also affect the timing and onset of puberty [22, 37, 39].

Many definitions for the timing of puberty exist in the literature, and this can cause confusion when examining the impact of factors such as obesity on the timing and tempo of puberty. The definition of puberty can be based on the shape of the adolescent growth spurt, the timing of sexual characteristics, specific events like menarche in girls and voice break in boys or skeletal maturation [18]. All of these factors likely contribute to the reported large variation in the timing of the onset of normal puberty.

While pubertal timing appears to be largely influenced by genetics, as implied by studies in twins [26], Karlberg suggests in his review from 2002 that a single environmental factor stands out as most significant – possibly explaining as much as 25% of the variation in the timing of puberty. This factor, it is stated, is simply the nutritional status in childhood – over-nutrition and obesity seem to trigger pubertal onset. However, recent studies have identified that both shortness and thinness at birth are also associated with earlier pubertal maturation – the reverse of their impact during childhood years [18]. Longitudinal series as opposed to cross-sectional series should be used to characterise the various pubertal events in more detail, thus providing more trustworthy information.

Effects of Puberty on Childhood Obesity Development

More than 2000 girls were examined in the 'National Health and Nutrition Examination Survey'. This survey consisted of a programme of studies that combined interviews and physical examinations to assess the health and nutritional status of adults and children in the USA. The mean age of menarche decreased by approximately 3 months in white girls and by 5.5 months in black girls in the USA between the late 1960s and approximately 1990, and this decrease was independent of weight. It is significant that the strongest evidence, i.e. the largest consistent changes, for the recent secular advancement of the onset and progression of puberty was found in the age at menarche for Mexican-American children and in black girls. These findings raise many questions concerning the definitions of race/ethnicity, concurrent secular changes in socioeconomic or health status, other USA minority populations, genetic potentials, and associations between changes in pubertal timing and obesity. In this study, the prevalence of early menarche was significantly increased if the girls had a BMI between the 85th and 95th percentile [17, 19]. Early pubertal development was also associated with a higher BMI and waist circumference in later life [40]. The studies in boys are less clear. One study investigated the effect of pubertal maturation and BMI on adipose tissue distribution and BMI during adulthood in 579 men [41, 42]. The age at the highest growth spurt correlated negatively with BMI, total body fat mass and central fat mass, but not with peripheral fat mass. An early start of pubertal development could therefore be a predictor for more centrally than peripherally increased fat mass in later life. A high amount of subcutaneous adipose tissue is rather a sign for a high BMI before puberty [42].

Obesity Influences Pubertal Development

Several studies on how childhood obesity can influence pubertal timing exist, but their results are sometimes controversial. The most important finding is that there are pronounced sex-dependent differences. A rapid weight gain during infancy (independent of birth weight) is associated with early pubertal development in both sexes. These data therefore support the hypothesis that fast body growth and rapid weight gain during infancy will influence pubertal development and induce earlier maturation [10].

Lue et al. found that a 1 unit (kg/m^2) greater BMI value at 8 years of age is associated with approximately a 1.3- and 1.2-month earlier age at peak height velocity for boys and girls, respectively [43]. Furthermore, results of a German study on 1,421 prepubertal children did not find significant differences in age when pubic hair was seen (of P2 Tanner) in lean and obese girls and boys. However, the age of thelarche was significantly earlier in obese girls, and an increase in testicular volume in boys appeared to be independent of BMI [44, 45].

In contrast, one study showed that childhood obesity could lead to a delayed timing of puberty. In 1,383 overweight and obese children, the following parameters were compared: body weight, height and timing of pubarche, menarche and voice break in a representative German childhood cohort aged 10–16 years [46]. Obese children were found to undergo later pubarche, menarche and voice break than their lean control group and hence presented with late puberty [46].

As described above, the study results are controversial. Therefore, it is of great importance to perform further and interdisciplinary studies to illuminate the connection between obesity and pubertal development and to better understand the sex-specific differences in these processes.

Childhood Obesity and Pubertal Development in Boys

Unfortunately, data about the connection between childhood obesity and pubertal development in boys is limited and controversial. Several studies have attempted to obtain significant and consistent data in relation to weight status and the timing and tempo of puberty [6, 22, 47–49].

One retrospective study included 1,520 men who were followed up until the age of 65. In this study, a high BMI during childhood was associated with an earlier timing of pubertal development [50], and children who showed late pubertal development were taller and leaner as adults. Furthermore, this study demonstrated that rapid weight gain during childhood resulted in early pubertal development and in shorter final height [50].

Another sign of pubertal maturation, the voice break, was evaluated in 436 choirboys from Denmark. The age at voice break decreased from 14.0 to 13.7 years within 10 years [51], and there was a trend towards an earlier voice break with increasing BMI [17, 41, 51].

Another puberty study from Copenhagen investigated the secular trend of pubertal timing in boys over a period of 15 years [47], comparing the pubertal timing during years 1991–1993 to that in 2006–2008. The researchers found that puberty, defined as a testis volume of >3 ml, started earlier in 2006–2008. Furthermore, the LH levels in this group were significantly increased compared to that of the first group, and the BMI-Standard Deviation Score (BMI-SDS) was found to be significantly higher in the second set of investigations. Interestingly, there were no significant differences in pubertal timing and serum LH levels during the two time frames after adjusting the BMI-SDS. In conclusion, this study found earlier pubertal development that seemed to be associated with increasing BMI [47].

The current data and publications on this topic are controversial; however, both hypotheses appear to be valid in that childhood obesity in boys can lead to an earlier or even delayed puberty. However, the majority of studies has shown that childhood obesity tends to be linked with an earlier timing of pubertal development in boys, but there are still too many inconsistencies to be able to answer the question properly. Further well-planned and interdisciplinary studies are needed to clarify these data.

Childhood Obesity and Pubertal Development in Girls

A large number of diverse studies have evaluated the connection between childhood obesity and pubertal development in girls. The results in girls, more strongly than those in boys, support the hypothesis that childhood obesity will lead to an earlier puberty onset. The major problem with these data is that they are mostly derived from cross-sectional studies; therefore, questions about the causality of this early onset of puberty remain unanswered. Girls that have a high BMI-SDS (>1.88) have a high probability of menstruating earlier, and they present with an earlier pubertal development than lean girls [44, 52–54]. Early puberty in girls can be caused by overweight and obesity, and this is definitely more often the case than puberty leading to a massive increase in body weight [55, 56].

Whether the general decrease in age for pubertal onset is a result of the so-called 'obesity epidemic' remains to be fully elucidated. A Danish study measured the age at puberty, the start of the pubertal growth spurt and the highest growth velocity of 156,835 pre-pubertal children [57]. In this study, the BMI-SDS correlated negatively with the parameters of pubertal development and pubertal timing. However, a trend towards an earlier puberty that is independent of BMI has been proven in the last 39 years, perhaps suggesting that the obesity epidemic is not the only reason for the secular trend towards earlier puberty that was seen in the 1900s [47, 57, 58].

Children who are small at birth and who develop obesity during childhood are significantly younger at the age of menarche than same-aged, lean children. In addition, the effect of maternal obesity on the pubertal development of daughters has not been investigated in depth [59]; however, one publication has indicated that daughters of mothers who were obese during pregnancy menstruate earlier than daughters of lean mothers [60].

In Switzerland, a longitudinal study examined 650 girls aged 6–18 years and did not find any significant differences in the ages of pubarche of lean and obese girls [61]. However, there were significant differences in the timing of breast development. Tanner stage B3 was reached at 11.6 years in obese girls compared to 12.2 years in normal-weight girls, and dehydroepiandrosterone levels were elevated [61].

The study data on girls is consistent and quite clear. However, the criticism is that most of the studies just looked at the outcome and did not determine the causes and reasons for earlier pubertal timing and development. How much influence does growth behaviours have on pubertal maturation? This question was studied using the mother and child files of the 'National Longitudinal Survey of Youth' [62]. In this study, significant differences in BMI and height at the age of 6 years in different ethnicities were found, which indicates that height and weight directly affect the age of menarche independent of derivation. These data are of enormous importance for understanding how height and weight differences influence the timing and maturation of puberty.

Molecular Mechanisms of Pubertal Onset

It has been known for many years that there is a close relationship between the reproductive axis and the amount and distribution of adipose tissue in girls. A female can only become pregnant if there is a sufficient amount of adipose tissue [63]. However, the molecular processes and mechanisms that link these systems remain unclear.

The relationship between childhood obesity and early puberty in girls could be explained by the insulin resistance/hyperinsulinaemia associated with obesity. In particular, increased insulin levels can stimulate sex steroid production by acting on adrenal glands, liver, ovary and fat cells. Increased androgen levels can in turn promote pubertal development by acting peripherally and/or centrally on the hypothalamic pituitary axis. With regards to GH-independent factors promoting growth, increased adipose tissue aromatisation of androgens into oestrogens is one of the main mechanisms that regulate growth in the context of obesity [12], and adrenal androgens seem to be an important mediator of adipose tissue and pubertal development. Whether adrenarche has a major impact on pubertal development has been discussed [12, 20]. One study examined lean and obese girls in Tanner stages 1–3 to identify clinical signs that are indicative of hyperandrogenaemia and to measure testosterone levels [64]. In obese girls, testosterone levels were elevated by 2–9×, and insulin levels were 3× higher than those of the lean control group. Peri-pubertal obesity seems to be associated with hyperandrogenaemia and hyperinsulinaemia during puberty. During the night, progesterone and testosterone levels increase in pubertal girls (Tanner stages 1–2), and this effect is more pronounced in obese girls [64]. Therefore, these data would suggest that high androgen levels in obese children in combination with elevated insulin levels could lead to earlier pubertal development in both sexes.

Genetic variance may also influence the processes of growth and pubertal development. For example, variations in the *LIN28B* gene have been shown to affect pubertal onset. Genetic variation of that gene could lead to an earlier thelarche in girls and to an earlier voice break and pubarche in boys [24, 26]. Furthermore, the pubertal growth spurt is reached early and the final height is reduced in those with genetic variation at this site. These data indicate that genetic factors might be a major link between the regulation of growth and pubertal development. In fact, they may be even more important than environmental factors.

There is also a clear secular trend in most developed countries towards increased height and weight, which affects the timing of puberty and onset of sexual activity [65]. Bruene et al. suggest that these changes have occurred too rapidly to invoke genetic modification as the causal factor. Instead, it is much more likely that epigenetic regulation of growth and maturational patterns, that is, developmental plasticity, has been decisive in this regard. This view is strongly supported by comparisons between populations that differ in nutritional supply, exposure to pathogens and socio-economic status [65].

Characteristics, like a low birth weight, early weight gain, early age at menarche and a smaller final height, are often found in several generations of females in one family. Genetic transmission has been proven to influence the age at menarche [59, 66–68], and pubertal development is very similar in twins, which is another sign of genetic determination [69]. One major point of criticism of most of the clinical studies cited in this article is that they have examined only children and adolescents during their development and have not taken into consideration information about the pubertal development and age at menarche of their parents, siblings or other relatives. Hence, this central factor has not been analysed in detail and needs to be further elucidated in future studies. So far, no genes have been identified that could be defined as pure 'puberty genes'. However, differences in chromosome 2 have been shown to be associated with late pubertal development, and one could speculate that there may be an internal clock in chromosome 2 that strongly influences the timing of pubertal onset [70].

Meta-analyses of genome-wide association studies have revealed that the following genes are associated with an early age of menarche: *TMEM38B*, *FKTN*, *FSD1L*, *TAL2*, *ZNF462* and *LIN28B* [26, 71]. Eleven genetic variations were found to be associated with an increased BMI, and five of those were correlated with a younger age at menarche [49]. These findings are all indications that genes may greatly influence both BMI and pubertal development.

Another important factor for pubertal onset and duration is the crosstalk between hormones, peptides from the gastrointestinal tract, adipose tissue and the central nervous system. Some factors can directly modulate the gonadotropic axis, and a lack of those peptides can lead to delayed timing of pubertal onset or to a slower progression of pubertal development. Several studies have defined leptin as a global player. It is known that BMI is positively associated with serum leptin levels and that leptin levels gradually rise with age prior to puberty in adolescents, suggesting a threshold effect that may trigger puberty [18]. Children who were shorter or thinner at pre-pubertal ages may experience a delayed tempo of development, as demonstrated by a younger bone age, thus slower skeleton maturation, and consequently, later timing of puberty [18]. Small amounts of leptin need to be administered to leptin-deficient mice to initialise pubertal onset, after which hypothalamic and pituitary gonadotropin secretion can be stimulated [13]. A study in rats showed that changes in the post-natal feeding period lead to effects on leptin and kisspeptin mRNA expression. Kisspeptin is thought to be a major regulator of puberty [72], and new findings suggest that leptin has a rather permissive role and that it is in fact not the main signal and regulator of puberty induction in children and adolescents. Therefore, several other factors must influence the energy balance, reproductive system and pubertal development, and there seems to be a complex interplay between these factors, of which many have probably still not been identified. Factors that may influence these systems are adiponectin and agouti-related peptide [4, 5, 7, 62]. In addition, ghrelin seems to also affect this complex system. Ghrelin is an orexigenic and growth-promoting peptide that is produced in the gastrointestinal tract, and ghrelin and other digestion peptides are believed to have a mediating role between energy homeostasis and sexual development [63, 73–75]. However, more studies are needed to further elucidate the exact role of these factors in pubertal development.

Over the last few years, the question as to whether endocrine-disrupting chemicals (EDCs) may be influencing pubertal development has been raised. Several studies from different countries have shown that EDCs affect pubertal onset [76], and in this context, there has also been proof of a strong migrative effect, which is also a sign that the environment influences that process [4]. At the moment, not enough studies have been performed in humans to draw final conclusions. The difficulty in making these conclusions is that many EDCs exist with heterogenous effects, and determining how to properly evaluate their effects on foetal and neonatal processes in humans is problematic. Research in animal models has clearly identified EDCs as factors that can influence pubertal onset and duration; however, the mechanisms remain unclear. New concepts support the hypothesis that EDCs are associated with a change in the energy balance and weight development [77].

The foetal and neonatal periods are important periods for the later development of growth, weight gain and pubertal onset. For example, girls that are born 'small for gestational age (SGA)', experience menarche on average 5 months earlier than girls with a normal birth weight, and a birth length that is 1 SDS (2 cm) lower than the average length is associated with an earlier peak growth velocity (about 1.3 months) [78–80]. The impact of intrauterine growth on the timing of puberty has been clearly observed, even after adjusting for length and BMI in childhood [43]. The long-term impact of foetal growth – such as its association with cardiovascular diseases – has been observed and has attracted much attention in recent years. It has been known that infants born SGA have much lower levels of neonatal and childhood serum leptin, insulin-like growth factor-I (IGF-1) and insulin-like growth factor binding protein-3. Karlberg speculates in his review that this subnormal neonatal hormone profile at birth may have a long-term imprinting effect on the post-natal timing of puberty, although the mechanism for this is unclear [18]. Peak height velocity in adolescence is reached at an earlier pubertal stage and lasts for a shorter period in children born SGA than in those born appropriate for gestational age. These differences lead to an earlier fusion of the growth plates and a shorter adult height. The pathophysiological mechanism underlying the unique pubertal growth pattern of children born SGA remains unclear; however, it seems that this is not only related to birth weight, gestational age, adiposity and obesity, but that rapid weight gain in early childhood may also influence pubertal onset. Excess weight gain in childhood may be related to central adiposity, decreased insulin sensitivity, and increased IGF-I levels and might thus predispose the individual to precocious pubarche [81]. Most importantly rapid and early weight gain during infancy increases the risk of being overweight or obese at the age of 5 and 8 (as demonstrated in the Avon Longitudinal Study of Parents and Children) [66]. Children with rapid and early weight gain often presented with insulin resistance, strong adrenarche and reduced sex hormone-binding globulin levels. One possible explanation for these occurrences is that obese children and adolescents have higher IGF-1 and androgen levels, which influence the activity of the enzyme aromatase. As a consequence, the concentrations of sexual steroids are increasing and the levels of sex hormone-binding globulin are decreasing, which can activate and increase the effect of the GnRH pulse generator [22]. Furthermore, increased leptin levels in obese children can initiate LH pulsatility [27]. One of the main risk factors for obesity and early menarche in girls is a rapid and early weight gain during infancy [17, 82]. However, the mechanisms that underlie those observations remain unclear, but researchers speculate that IGF-1 could be a major player.

Psychological Aspects of Childhood Obesity and Early Pubertal Development

Earlier onset of puberty is a strong psychological burden for girls and boys. Children and adolescents are often teased when they experience an early development of thelarche and pubarche compared to girls and boys at the same age. Obese boys who have to cope with lipogynaecomastia often suffer the most. One study from Boston describes the negative effects of lipogynaecomastia on quality of life and self esteem as well as the psychological symptoms and the aftermath of eating behaviours. The results from this study were even independent of BMI [83]. Occasionally, eating disorders are the underlying reason for obesity. For example, 'binge eating' leads to a reduced quality of life and is associated with low self-esteem, and subsequent problems with social interactions will lead to solitude [84]. These results are from studies that have either looked at the psychological aspects of early pubertal development or from studies that evaluated the psychological effects of obesity during childhood and adolescence. Rarely, these studies have combined and investigated both problems at once, although many adolescents have to cope with both difficulties and will therefore experience more psychological distress.

Comorbidities and Consequences of Childhood Obesity and Early Pubertal Development

One of the long-term consequences of obesity and early pubertal onset is a higher risk for cancer development during adulthood [85]. An early menarche is a risk factor for the development of breast cancer in females [86, 87]. Another problem is that girls who suffer from an earlier puberty usually need to become 'adults and be grown-up' earlier and are generally sexually active at a younger age, although they still often show immature childhood behaviours. Whether there are also negative effects of early puberty on fertility needs to be elucidated in the future.

Obesity during puberty in girls often leads to hyperandrogenaemia and a higher risk for the development of polycystic ovaries [64], which are often associated with fertility problems later in life. Associated insulin resistance and hyperinsulinaemia will influence other hormone levels and will therefore also adversely affect pubertal development.

Childhood obesity can be associated with several metabolic and cardiovascular complications during childhood and adolescence. Metabolic syndrome is not only a disease of later life; obese children already present symptoms of metabolic syndrome, including insulin resistance, impaired glucose tolerance, high levels of triglycerides and arterial hypertonus [29]. Whether the earlier timing of puberty in combination with childhood obesity aggravates metabolic and cardiovascular comorbidities needs to be elucidated in new, well-planned and interdisciplinary studies.

Childhood obesity in combination with early pubertal onset can lead to various psychosocial and physical problems that will negatively impact and reduce life quality and expectancy.

Summary/Conclusion

Studies have shown that there is a clear relationship between reaching a critical body weight and pubertal onset and course. Moreover, rapid and early weight gain during infancy and even during foetal life is associated with early onset of menarche, an early pubertal growth spurt, early thelarche in girls, earlier pubarche in both sexes and an earlier increase in testicular volume in boys. The early onset of puberty could be mediated through factors that are directly linked to adipose tissue (e.g. adipocytokines) or might be an indirect effect of genetic and/or environmental factors (e.g. genes, EDCs or social environment). From an evolutionary point of view, not every pubertal development process is associated with advantageous reproductive competence. On the contrary, early puberty is an immense psychological and social disadvantage that affects the reproductive system and likely the cardiovascular and metabolic health of the affected individuals [16, 22, 77].

Due to the inconsistencies in the data, we suggest the initiation of new and interdisciplinary studies that address the problem in more detail and that further evaluate the possible underlying mechanisms. Afterward, we should readdress the question of whether obesity influences pubertal development in both sexes to the same degree and try to identify the factors that link adipose tissue to the pubertal-gonadal axis.

Literature Search

PubMed was used for a systematic literature search for articles in English and German that were published until the end of 2013; the main focus was on articles from the last 10 years. The following key words were used: *'puberty and obesity', 'body mass index', 'peak height velocity', 'menarche', 'pubic hair stage', 'puberty', 'secular trend', 'boys', 'girls'*. The references in those articles were analysed, and the data and summaries have been thoroughly evaluated by the authors.

References

1 Frisch RE, Revelle R: Height and weight at menarche and a hypothesis of critical body weights and adolescent events. Science 1970;169:397–399.

2 Johnston FE, Malina RM, Galbraith MA, Frisch RE, Revelle R, Cook S: Height, weight and age at menarche and the 'critical weight' hypothesis. Science 1971;174:1148–1149.

3 Frisch RE: Pubertal adipose tissue: Is it necessary for normal sexual maturation? Evidence from the rat and human female. Fed Proc 1980;39:2395–2400.

4 Parent AS, Teilmann G, Juul A, Skakkebaek NE, Toppari J, Bourguignon JP: The timing of normal puberty and the age limits of sexual precocity: variations around the world, secular trends, and changes after migration. Endocr Rev 2003;24:668–693.

5 de Muinck Keizer-Schrama SMPF, Mul D: Trends in pubertal development in Europe. Hum Reprod Update 2001;7:287–291.

6 Mul D, Frederiks AM, van Buuren S, Oostdijk W, Verloove-Vanhorick SP, Wit JM: Pubertal development in The Netherlands. Pediatr Res 2001;50:479–486.

7 Bourguignon JP, Rasier G, Lebrethon MC, Gerard A, Naveau E, Parent AS: Neuroendocrine disruption of pubertal timing and interactions between homeostasis of reproduction and energy balance. Mol Cell Endocrinol 2010;324:110–120.

8 Freedman DS, Khan LK, Serdula MK, Dietz WH, Srinivasan SR, Berenson GS: Relation of age at menarche to race, time period, and anthropometric dimensions: The Bogalusa Heart Study. Pediatrics 2002;110:e34.

9 Papadimitriou A: Sex differences in the secular changes in pubertal maturation. Pediatrics 2001; 108:e65.

10 Boyne MS, Thame M, Osmond C, Fraser RA, Gabay L, Reid M, Forrester TE: Growth, body composition, and the onset of puberty: longitudinal observations in Afro-Caribbean children. J Clin Endocrinol Metab 2010;95:3194–3200.

11 Turi KN, Christoph MJ, Grigsby-Toussaint DS: Spatial distribution of underweight, overweight among women and children. Results from the 2011 Uganda demographic and health survey. Int J Environ Res Public Health 2013;10:4967–4981.

12 Marcovecchio ML, Chiarelli F: Obesity and growth during childhood and puberty. World Rev Nutr Diet 2013;106:135–141.

13 Kiess W, Müller G, Galler A, Reich A, Detscher J, Klammt J, Kratzsch J: Body fat mass, leptin and puberty. J Pediatr Endocrinol Metab 2000;13:(suppl 1): 717–722.

14 Kiess W, Reich A, Meyer K, Glasow A, Deutscher J, Klammt J, Yang Y, Müller G, Kratsch J: A role for leptin in sexual maturation and puberty? Horm Res 1999;51:55–63.

15 Han JC, Lawlor DA, Kimm SYS: Childhood obesity. Lancet 2010;375:1737–1748.

16 Solorzano CM, Mc Cartney CR: Obesity and the pubertal transition in girls and boys. Reproduction 2010;140:399–410.

17 Ong KK, Emmett P, Northstone K, Golding J, Rogers I, Ness AR, Wells JC, Dunger DB: Infancy weight gain predicts childhood body fat and age at menarche in girls. J Clin Endocrinol Metab 2009;94: 1527–1532.

18 Karlberg J: Secular trends in pubertal development. Horm Res 2002;57:19–30.

19 Himes JH: Examining the evidence for recent secular changes in the timing of puberty in US children in light of increases in the prevalence of obesity. Mol Cell Endocrinol 2006;254-255:13–21

20 Himes JP, Park K, Styne D: Menarche and assessment of body mass index in adolescent girls. J Pediatr 2009;155:393–397.

21 Blüher S, Meigen C, Gausche R, Keller E, Pfäffle R, Sabin M, Werther G, Odeh R, Kiess W: Age-specific stabilization in obesity prevalence in German children: a cross-sectional study from 1999 to 2008. Int J Pediatr Obes 2011;6:199–206.

22 Wagner IV, Sabin MA, Pfäffle RW, Hiemisch A, Sergeyev E, Körner A, Kiess W: Effects of obesity on human sexual development. Nat Rev Endocrinol 2012; 8:246–254.

23 Christakis NA, Fowler JH: The spread of obesity in a large social network over 32 years. New Engl J Med 2007;357:370–379.
24 Tommiska J, Wehkalampi K, Vaaralahti K, Laitinen EM, Raivio T, Dunkel L: LIN28B in constitutional delay of growth and puberty. J Clin Endocrinol Metab 2010;95:3063–3066.
25 Körner A, Ma L, Franks PB, Kiess W, Baier LJ, Stumvoll M, Kovacs P: Gender specific effect of the Val-1483Ile polymorphism in the fatty acid synthase gene (FAS) on body mass index and lipid profile in Caucasian children. Int J Obes 2007;31:353–358.
26 Ong KK, Elks CE, Li S, Zhao JH, Luan J, Barroso I, Mooser V, Loos RJ, Wareham NJ: Genetic variation in LIN28B is associated with the timing of puberty. Nat Genet 2009;41:729–733
27 Fraser AK, Macdonald-Wallis C, Sattar N, Brion MJ, Benfield L, Ness A, Deanfield J, Hingorani A, Nelson SM, Smith GD, Lawlor DA: Association of maternal weight gain in pregnancy with offspring obesity and metabolic and vascular traits in childhood. Circulation 2010;121:2557–2564
28 Fredriks AM, van Buuren S, Burgmeijer RJ, Meulmeester JF, Beuker RJ, Brugman E, Roede MJ, Verloove-Vanhorick SP, Wit JM: Continuing positive secular growth change in The Netherlands 1955–1997. Pediatr Res 2000;47:316–323.
29 Kiess W, Blüher S, Kapellen T, Körner A: Metabolic syndrome in children and adolescents: prevalence, public health issue, and time for initiative. J Pediatr Gastroenterol Nutr 2009;49:268–71.
30 Sharma M: International school-based interventions for preventing obesity in children. Obes Rev 2007;8: 155–167.
31 Körner A, Kratzsch J, Gausche R, Schaab M, Erbs S, Kiess W: New predictors of the metabolic syndrome in children – role of adipocytokines. Pediatr Res 2007;61:640–645
32 Körner A, Kiess W, Stumvoll M, Kovacs P: Polygenic contribution to obesity: genome-wide strategies reveal new targets. Frontiers of hormone research. 2008;36:12–36.
33 Wiegand S, Maikowski U, Blankenstein O, Biebermann H, Tarnow P, Grüters A: Type 2 diabetes and impaired glucose tolerance in European children and adolescents with obesity – a problem that is no longer restricted to minority groups. Eur J Endocrinol 2004;151:199–206.
34 Sinha R, Fisch G, Teague B, Tamborlane WV, Banyas B, Allen K, Savoye M, Rieger V, Taksali S, Barbette G, Sherwin RS, Caprio S: Prevalence of impaired glucose tolerance among children and adolescents with marked obesity. New Engl J Med 2002;346:802–810.
35 Reich A, Müller G, Gelbrich G, Deutscher K, Gödicke R, Kiess W: Obesity and blood pressure – results from the examination of 2365 schoolchildren in Germany. Int J Obes 2003;27:1459–1464.
36 Kiess W, Galler A, Reich A, Müller G, Kapellen T, Deutscher J, Raile K, Kratzsch J: Clinical aspects of obesity in childhood and adolescence. Obes Rev 2001;2:29–36.
37 DiVall SA, Radovick S: Endocrinology of female puberty. Curr Opin Endocrinol Diabetes Obes 2009;16: 1–4.
38 Delemarre-van de Waal HA: Regulation of puberty. Best Pract Res Clin Endocrinol Metab 2002;16:1–12.
39 Rosenfield RL, Cooke DW, Radovick S: Puberty and its disorder in the female; in Sperling MA (ed): Pediatric Endocrinology, ed 3. Philadelphia, PA, Saunders/Elsevier, 2008, pp 565–569.
40 Ogden C, Carroll M: Prevalence of Obesity Among Children and Adolescents: United States, Trends 1963–1965 Through 2007—2008. Healthy People, National Center for Health Statistics, Division of Health and Nutrition Examination Surveys, 2010.
41 Kindblom JM, Lorentzon M, Norjavaara E, Hellqvist A, Nilsson S, Mellström D, Ohlsson C: Pubertal timing predicts previous fractures and BMD in young adult men: the GOOD study. J Bone Miner Res 2006; 21:790–795.
42 Kindblom JM, Lorentzon M, Norjavaara E, Lönn L, Brandberg J, Angelhed JE, Hellqvist A, Nilsson S, Ohlsson C: Pubertal timing is an independent predictor of central adiposity in young adult males: the Gothenburg osteoporosis and obesity determinants study. Diabetes 2006;55:3047–3052.
43 Luo ZC, Cheung YB, He Q, Albertsson-Wikland K, Karlberg J: Growth in early life and its relation to pubertal growth. Epidemiology 2003;14:65–73.
44 Heger S, Körner A, Meigen C, Gausche R, Keller A, Keller E, Kiess W: Impact of weight status on the onset and parameters of puberty: analysis of three representative cohorts from central Europe. J Pediatr Endocrinol Metab 2008;21:865–877.
45 Meigen C, Keller A, Gausche R, Kronmeyer-Hausschild K, Blüher S, Kiess W, Keller E: Secular trends in body mass index in German children and adolescents: a cross-sectional data analysis via CrescNet between 1999 and 2006. Metabolism 2008;7:934–949.
46 Kleber M, Schwarz A, Reinehr T: Obesity in children and adolescents: relationship to growth, pubarche, menarche, and voice break. J Pediatr Endocrinolo Metab 2011;24:125–130.
47 Sørensen K, Aksglaede L, Petersen JH, Juul A: Recent changes in pubertal timing in healthy Danish boys: associations with body mass index. J Clin Endocrinol Metab 2010;95:263–270.

48 de Onis M, Dasgupta P, Saha S, Sengupta D, Blossner M: The National Center for Health Statistics reference and the growth of Indian adolescent boys. Amer J Clin Nutrition 2001;74:248–253.
49 Sulem P, Gudbjartsson DF, Rafnar T, Holm H, Olafsdottir EJ, Tryggvadottir L, Thorsteindottir U, Stefansson K: Genome-wide association study identifies sequence variants on 6q21 associated with age at menarche. Nat Genet 2009;41:734–738.
50 Sandhu J, Ben Shlomo Y, Cole TJ, Holly J, Davey SG: The impact of childhood body mass index on timing of puberty, adult stature and obesity: a follow-up study based on adolescent anthropometry recorded at Christ's Hospital (1936–1964). Int J Obes (Lond) 2006;30:14–22.
51 Juul A, Magnusdottir S, Scheike T, Prytz S, Skakkebaek NE: Age at voice break in Danish boys: effects of pre-pubertal body mass index and secular trend. Int J Androl 2007;30:537–542.
52 Wang Y: Is obesity associated with early sexual maturation? A comparison of the association in American boys versus girls. Pediatrics 2004;113:171–172.
53 Kaplowitz PB, Slora EJ, Wasserman RC, Pedlow SE, Herman-Giddens ME: Earlier onset of puberty in girls: relation to increased body mass index and race. Pediatrics. 2001;108:347–353.
54 Kirchengast S, Bauer M: Menarcheal onset is associated with body composition parameters but not with socioeconomic status. Coll Antropol 2007;31:419–425.
55 Biro FM, Huang B, Morrison JA, Horn PS, Daniels SR: Body mass index and waist-to-height changes during teen years in girls are influenced by childhood body mass index. J Adolesc Health 2010;46: 245–250.
56 Biro FM, Khoury P, Morrison JA: Influence of obesity on timing of puberty. Int J Androl 2006;29:272–277.
57 Aksglaede L, Juul A, Olsen LW, Sørensen TI: Age at puberty and the emerging obesity epidemic. PLoS One 2009;4:e8450.
58 Aksglaede L, Sorensen K, Petersen JH, Skakkebaek NE, Juul A: Recent decline in age at breast development: the Copenhagen Puberty Study. Pediatrics 2009;123:e932–e939
59 Ibáñez L, Lopez-Bermejo A, Diaz M, Marcos MV, de Zegher F: Early metformin therapy to delay menarche and augment height in girls with precocious pubarche. Fertil Steril 2011;95:727–730
60 Keim SA, Branum AM, Klebanoff MA, Zemel BS: Maternal body mass index and daughters' age at menarche. Epidemiology 2009;20:677–681.
61 Prader A, Largo RH, Molinari L, Issler C: Physical growth of Swiss children from birth to 20 years of age. First Zurich longitudinal study of growth and development. Helv Paediatr Acta Suppl 1989;52:1–125.
62 Salsberry PJ, Reagan PB, Pajer K: Growth differences by age of menarche in African American and White girls. Nurs Res 2009;58:382–390.
63 Martos-Moreno GA, Chowen JA, Argente J: Metabolic signals in human puberty: effects of over and undernutrition. Mol Cell Endocrinol 2010;324:70–81.
64 McCartney CR, Blank SK, Prendergast KA, Chhabra S, Eagleson CA, Helm KD, Yoo R, Chang RJ, Foster CM, Caprio S, Marshall JC: Obesity and sex steroid changes across puberty: evidence for marked hyperandrogenemia in pre- and early pubertal obese girls. J Clin Endocrinol Metab 2007;92:430–436.
65 Bruene M, Hochberg Z: Secular trends in new childhood epidemics: insights from evolutionary medicine. BMC Med 2013;11:226.
66 Dunger DB, Ahmed ML, Ong KK: Early and late weight gain and the timing of puberty. Mol Cell Endocrinol 2006;254–255:140–145.
67 Gluckman PD, Hanson MA: Evolution, development and timing of puberty Trends Endocrinol Metab 2006;17:7–12.
68 Papadimitriou A, Nicolaidou P, Fretzayas A, Chrousos GP: Clinical review: constitutional advancement of growth acceleration, predicts early puberty and childhood obesity. J Clin Endocrinol Metab 2010;95: 4535–4541.
69 Hoekstra RA, Bartels M, Boomsma DI: Heritability of testosterone levels in 12-year-old twins and its relation to pubertal development. Twin Res Hum Genet 2006;9:558–565.
70 Wehkalampi K, Widén E, Laine T, Palotie A, Dunkel L: Association of the timing of puberty with a chromosome 2 locus. J Clin Endocrinol Metab 2008;93: 4833–4839.
71 Perry JRB, Stolk L, Franceschine N, Lunettea KL, Zhai G, Mc Ardke PF, Demerath EW, Uitterlinden AG, Murabito JM: Meta-analysis of genome-wide association data identifies two loci influencing age at menarche. Nat Genet 2009;41:648–650.
72 Castellano JM, Bentsen AH, Sánchez-Garrido MA, Ruiz-Pino F, Romero M, Garcia-Galiano D, Aguilar E, Pinilla L, Diéguez C, Mikkelsen JD, Tena-Sempere M: Early metabolic programming of puberty onset: impact of changes in postnatal feeding and rearing conditions on the timing of puberty and development of the hypothalamic kisspeptin system. Endocrinology 2011;152:3396–3408.
73 Whatmore AJ, Hall CM, Jones J, Westwood M, Clayton PE: Ghrelin concentrations in healthy children and adolescents. Clin Endocrinol 2003;59:649–654.
74 Pomerants T, Tillmann V, Jürimäe J, Jürimäe T: Relationship between ghrelin and anthropometrical, body composition parameters and testosterone levels in boys at different stages of puberty. J Endocrinol Invest 2006;29:962–967.

75 Ebbeling CB, Pawlak DB, Ludwig DS: Childhood obesity: public-health crisis, common sense cure. Lancet 2002;360:473–482.
76 Özen S, Darcon Ş: Effects of environmental endocrine disruptors on pubertal development. J Clin Res Pediatr Endocrinol 2011;3:1–6.
77 Diamanti-Kandarakis E, Bourguignon JP, Giudice LC, Hauser R, Prins GS, Soto AM, Zoeller RT, Gore AC: Endocrine-disrupting chemicals: an Endocrine Society scientific statement. Endocr Rev 2009;30: 293–342.
78 Ferrer A, Marcos MV, Hierro FR, de Zegher F: Early puberty: rapid progression and reduced final height in girls with low birth weight. Pediatrics 2000;106: e72.
79 Adair LS: Size at birth predicts age at menarche. Pediatrics 2011;107:e59.
80 Tam CS, de Zegher F, Garnett SP, Baur LA, Cowell CT: Opposing influences of prenatal and postnatal growth on the timing of menarche. J Clin Endocrinol Metab 2006;91:4369–4373.
81 Verkauskiene R, Petraitiene I, Albertsson Wikland K: Puberty in children born small for gestational age. Horm Res Peadiatr 2013;80:69–77.
82 Ong KK, Langkamp M, Ranke MB, Whitehead K, Hughes IA, Acerini CL, Dunger DB: Insulin-like growth factor I concentrations in infancy predict differential gains in body length and adiposity: the Cambridge Baby Growth Study. Am J Clin Nutr 2009;90:156–161.
83 Cerrato F, Webb ML, Rosen H, Nuzzi L, Mc Carty ER, Di Vasta AD, Greene AK, Labow BI: The impact of macromastia on adolescents: a cross-sectional study. Pediatrics 2012;339–346.
84 Ranzenhofer LM, Columbo KM, Tanofsky-Kraff M, Shomaker LB, Cassidy O, Metheson BE, Kolotkin RL, Checchi JM, Keil M, Mc Duffie JR, Yanovski JA: Binge eating and weight-related quality of life in obese adolescents. Nutrients 2012;4:167–180.
85 Gilbert CA, Slingerland JM: Cytokines, obesity, and cancer: new insights on mechanisms linking obesity to cancer risk and progression. Annu Rev Med 2013; 64:45–57.
86 Apter D, Vihko R: Early menarche, a risk factor for breast cancer, indicates early onset of ovulatory cycles. J Clin Endocrinol Metab 1983;57:82–86.
87 Vihko RK, Apter DL: The epidemiology and endocrinology of the menarche in relation to breast cancer. Cancer Szrv 1986;5:561–571.

Prof. Wieland Kiess, MD
Department of Women and Child Health
Hospital for Children and Adolescents, University of Leipzig
Liebigstrasse 20a
DE–04103 Leipzig (Germany)
E-Mail wieland.kiess@medizin.uni-leipzig.de

Kiess W, Wabitsch M, Maffeis C, Sharma AM (eds): Metabolic Syndrome and Obesity in Childhood and Adolescence.
Pediatr Adolesc Med. Basel, Karger, 2015, vol 19, pp 126–136 (DOI: 10.1159/000368113)

Urban Living Conditions: The Relation between Neighborhood Characteristics and Obesity in Children and Adolescents

Ulrike Igel · Gesine Grande

Faculty of Architecture and Social Sciences, Leipzig University of Applied Sciences (HTWK Leipzig), Leipzig, Germany

Abstract

The individual risks for obesity have been studied extensively. Therefore, this chapter focuses on environmental conditions that promote unhealthy weight gain in children and adolescents. Beginning with a theoretical conceptualization of what constitutes a neighborhood, we report on recent findings on compositional (e.g. area socioeconomic deprivation), structural (e.g. physical environment, i.e. the availability of parks and facilities for physical activity), and functional (e.g. social environment, i.e. social capital and social cohesion within a neighborhood) aspects of neighborhoods and their impact on obesity in children and adolescents. In the following section, we describe the theoretical models of differing complexity that are used to explain spatial effects on child health. In the concluding section, findings and methods are discussed, and implications for community-based obesity prevention are proposed.

Introduction

This chapter takes a different perspective on metabolic syndrome and obesity by focusing on the environmental determinants and the potential influence of the urban environment and living conditions on obesity in children and adolescents. Traditionally, research has focused on individual characteristics (e.g. lifestyle, family socioeconomic status, currently also genetics), and this has led to an imbalance between research on individual and environmental risks [1]. As Diez Roux et al. [2] stated, there are at least four reasons for taking the environment into account: (1) individual characteristics are insufficient for explaining health (behavior), (2) health inequalities cannot be adequately explained by individual risks, (3) there is increasing availability of more sophisticated methods to analyze the impact of environmental factors on health outcomes (multi-level analyses, Geographic Information Systems), and (4) prevention efforts need to consider policy aspects that are implemented in the contexts in which individuals live.

Environment or Neighborhood: An Attempt at a Definition

A considerable body of research has investigated environmental influences on health. However, there is extensive discussion about how to define and measure the 'environment' [3]. The selection of environmental variables as well as their designation depends on the scientific provenience of the researchers, the country where the study is carried out, and the available data. A large number of studies on the environmental influences on health outcomes have applied the term 'neighborhood'; therefore, we use this term as a synonym for community, spatial unit, residence, and place. According to the definition proposed by Earls and Carlson, neighborhoods are a set of social relationships that may be historically established by different types of social or political interests and can be 'defined and measured in terms of their composition, structure and function' [4]. Composition refers to the sociodemographic characteristics of the residents; structure comprises social and physical arrangements (institutions, built/physical environment) that are beyond an individual's control and may facilitate or constrain the daily activities of the residents; and function implies the quality of interactions as well as the degree of shared values and expectations (e.g. social environment or 'collective social functioning') [4]. Although this definition is useful for explaining the 'content' or components of neighborhoods, it neglects the interdependence (interaction) of all of these dimensions as well as the physical boundaries of neighborhoods. There is an ongoing debate in public health research regarding how to spatially define neighborhoods or 'places' [5]. Traditionally, individuals' addresses were linked to the corresponding administrative area (e.g. census tracts) where data on aggregate socioeconomic status were already available. With the increasing involvement of geographers in public health research and the growing popularity of Geographic Information Systems, more sophisticated methods have been developed to analyze the 'individual' environment of a person. For example, buffer zones around a child's home or school have been created to capture aspects of the physical environment within a certain spatial unit [3]. However, these approaches are quite conventional and neglect an individual's mobility as well as changes in individuals and places over time. Currently, some researchers have proposed a relational view, which defines neighborhoods or areas in a relatively dynamic and fluid manner and takes into account individual and spatial changes over time [5]. Both approaches are valuable. The conventional definition is useful and appropriate for public health agents evaluating the health-related aspects of certain administrative areas in order to develop adequate interventions for a particular region rather than for a single person. The relational view seems to be more appropriate for explaining and understanding place effects by capturing an individual's 'real' action space or areas of potential influences.

The Obesogenic Environment? Evidence of Neighborhood Effects on Childhood Obesity

Since the late nineties, the term 'obesogenic environment' has been defined as 'the sum of influences that the surroundings, opportunities, or conditions of life have on promoting obesity in individuals or populations' [6]. The core questions are as follows: Are individuals living in neighborhood A more likely to become obese than those living in neighborhood B? Are there obesogenic environments, and what are they like? The influencing factors have been investigated in reference to the composition (socioeconomic status, deprivation), structure (physical environment), and function (social environment) of neighborhoods. In the following sections, the findings are illustrated by drawing on recent reviews of environmental influences on obesity in children and adolescents [3, 7–9].

Composition: Area-Level Socioeconomic Status or Deprivation
Traditionally, the compositional effect of neighborhoods on obesity in children and adolescents has been studied by investigating the aggregate socioeconomic status (SES) or deprivation of neighborhoods using official data from administrative spatial units (e.g. census tracts, school districts). SES at the area level is commonly measured using one or more of the following indicators: unemployment rate, median income, proportion of educational levels, single parents, and material possessions (such as a private car and central heating in the house). Some studies have used composite indices (e.g. Townsend deprivation index, Carstairs index, Index of multiple deprivation), whereas others have included single variables. Based on three reviews on neighborhood deprivation (or SES) and childhood obesity, the majority of the studies have reported associations between neighborhood deprivation and overweight or obesity in children and adolescents [3, 8, 9]. The evidence has suggested that increased neighborhood disadvantage (or low neighborhood socioeconomic status) is related to an increased prevalence of obesity. However, other studies have found no significant associations.

Structure: Physical Environment
Since the late nineties, questions about the structural aspects of environments and their effects on obesity have become more popular. These structural aspects are often referred to as the 'physical environment', which comprises aspects of infrastructure and of the built and natural environment as well as services (institutions) that are provided publicly or privately [10]. Measurements of the physical environment usually include features such as green space and parks, playgrounds and sports or recreational facilities,

and characteristics of walkability (e.g. street connectivity, dwelling density, land-use mix). The findings on the influences of these factors on obesity in children and adolescents have been inconsistent; however, there is some evidence that the proportion of green space is negatively related to obesity in children. Other studies have found no association between the number of and distance to parks and obesity. The availability of sports and recreational facilities and playgrounds tends to be related to obesity and body mass index. Four of seven studies reviewed by Carter and Dubois [3] and Dunton et al. [7] reported a negative association between the number and accessibility of facilities for physical activity (e.g. playgrounds, sports and recreational facilities) and obesity in children, whereas in two of the studies, the association was significant only in girls. Concerning the influence of walkability on childhood obesity, there is little evidence, and most of the reviewed studies have found no associations. Only Spence et al. [11] found that walkability characteristics (e.g. dwelling density, land-use-mix, and intersection density) were negatively related to overweight in girls [3, 7].

Function: Social Environment
The functional aspects of neighborhoods are often referred to as the 'social environment.' These aspects are usually measured by perceived social cohesion, social capital, collective socialization, and social control as well as parents' or adolescents' perceptions of safety. Whereas the association between safety and childhood obesity has been reasonably well studied (showing no relation, with the exception of road safety) [3], studies on the relation between the social environment, defined as social capital, cohesion, trust, etc., and childhood obesity are still scarce. However, when investigating a neighborhood's social capital, social cohesion, or trust, negative associations with obesity in children and adolescents could be found.

The findings of the opening questions of whether there are 'obesogenic environments' and what are they like are ambiguous. Regarding compositional aspects of a neighborhood, i.e. socioeconomic status or deprivation, associations with obesity in children and adolescents have been extensively studied and are evident. Children and adolescents living in deprived neighborhoods are at higher risk of becoming obese. In relation to aspects of the physical environment, there is some evidence to suggest that obesity and the amount of green space and the availability of facilities are associated, but the findings are conflicting. Children and adolescents living in neighborhoods with a small proportion of green space and few available sports and recreational facilities (including playgrounds) may be more likely to become obese. Concerning the functional aspects of neighborhoods, only characteristics drawing on the quality of social relations (e.g. social capital, social cohesion, and trust) have been found to be associated with obesity in children and adolescents, but such studies are still scarce. Children and adolescents living in neighborhoods with low social capital and low social cohesion may be more likely to become obese. The summary of the reviewed studies [3, 7–9, 12], shown in table 1, is *not* exhaustive, but it reflects the inconsistencies in the findings.

Table 1. Studies on associations between urban conditions and childhood obesity

Socioeconomic status/deprivation		Greenness, parks		Facilities		Walkability		Social environment	
Association	No association	Association	No association	Association	No association	Association	No association	Association	No association
Chen and Paterson [25], 2006	Janssen et al. [26], 2006	Bell et al. [49], 2008	Norman et al. [51], 2006	Veugelers et al. [29], 2008	Burdette and Whitaker [55], 2004	(Spence et al. [11], 2008)	Grafova [30], 2008	McKay et al. [58], 2007	*Burdette and Whitaker* [59], *2005*
Janssen et al. [26], 2006	Janssen et al. [26], 2006	Liu et al. [50], 2007	Kligerman et al. [52], 2006	Gordon-Larsen et al. [53], 2006	Timperio et al. [56], 2005		Spence et al. [11], 2008	Veitch et al. [12], 2012	*Lumeng et al.* [60], *2006*
Koller and Mielck [27], 2009	Koller and Mielck [27], 2009		(Scott et al.) [39], 2007	(Evenson et al.) [54], 2007			Merchant et al. [57], 2007	*Timperio et al.* [57], *2005*	*O'Brien et al.* [61], *2007*
Oliver and Hayes [28], 2008	Wright [43], 2004			(Spence et al.) [11], 2008			Norman et al. [51], 2006		*Veugelers et al.* [29], *2008*
Veugelers et al. [29], 2008	Cohen et al. [44], 2006						Kligerman et al. [52], 2006		*Evenson et al.* [54], *2007*
Grafova [30], 2008	Brunt et al. [45], 2008								
Kinra et al. [31], 2000	Dummer et al. [46], 2005								
Oliver and Hayes, [32], 2005	Burke et al. [47], 2004								
Cecil et al. [33], 2005	Cowell et al. [48], 1999								
Rutter [34], 2008									
Emerson [35], 2009									
Armstrong et al. [36], 2003									
Wardle et al. [37], 2006									
Jansen and Hazebroek-Kampschreur [38], 1997									
(Scott et al.) [39], 2007									
(Sweeting et al.) [40], 2008									
(Wardle et al.) [41], 2003									
(Booth et al.) [42], 1999									

( ) only in subgroups (females); *italics* = safety.

Why and How Does the Neighborhood Contribute to Obesity in Children and Adolescents? Causes and Mechanisms

There is general agreement that environment matters, but little evidence as to why and how exactly it influences health outcomes is available. Identifying statistically relevant neighborhood characteristics does not mean that we understand the mechanisms and pathways behind the analysis. There are different conceptual frameworks that generally explain, in a more or less complex way, the associations between the environment and well-being of a child and that may also be useful for clarifying the pathways between neighborhood characteristics and obesity.

Compositional Versus Contextual Explanations

Early attempts to answer the question of why health risks are spatially patterned led to the distinction between compositional and contextual explanations [10, 13]. The compositional explanation ascribes spatial differences in health outcomes to an accumulation of individuals with similar characteristics in particular places [10]. For example, children in deprived areas are less physically active because their parents cannot afford the fees for organized sports or do not have the resources to take them to parks, etc., which means that the spatial effect is a consequence of only the spatial concentration of socioeconomically deprived or advantaged people in different areas [13]. Contextual explanations attribute spatial differences in health outcomes to characteristics of the physical and social environment that are beyond the individual's control, e.g. the availability or absence of resources such as recreational facilities and institutions but also social norms and relations. For example, children in deprived areas are less physically active because only a few facilities (parks, sports facilities) are provided in the area. Moreover, physical activity may not be seen as something important for children within the local culture [10]. This distinction has been criticized because it oversimplifies the underlying mechanisms and social realities by neglecting interactions between people and places, and it is impossible to demonstrate this distinction empirically [14].

Direct-Effect Structural Models Versus Indirect-Effect Models

Other attempts to understand the spatial effects on child health can be seen in direct-effect structural models and indirect-effect models, which comprise compositional and contextual perspectives.

Based on a rather psychological perspective, Jencks and Mayer [15] developed theoretical models that provide an explanation of the consequences of aggregate poverty (i.e. neighborhood deprivation). These models can be considered to be 'direct-effect structural models' because the structures of a child's physical and social environment are directly linked to her health [16, 17]. By employing the theoretical frameworks but without explaining every single model, we present some examples of how children or adolescents growing up in deprived neighborhoods might become overweight or obese.

Living in a deprived neighborhood might be related to the following.

- A lack of resources (e.g. parks, recreational facilities for physical activities) that provide healthy learning and living environments (institutional resource model) [15, 18].
- A decrease in formal and informal institutions (e.g. adults, schools 'controlling' health behavior) that supervise and monitor the children's behaviors (collective socialization model) [15, 18].
- A spread of behavioral problems or unhealthy behavior in peers, e.g. fast food consumption, physical inactivity but also shared values and perceptions of body shape (epidemic model) [15, 18].

Other efforts have been made to distinguish the possible influencing factors by emphasizing four pathways: (1) differences in the availability and quality of neighborhood institutions and resources (especially health care facilities and transportation), (2) stress factors in the physical environment (e.g. poorly maintained facilities for physical activity), (3) stress factors in the social environment (in particular, crime) that may hinder health-promoting behavior, and (4) social networks and norms that shape health-related behavior [17].

These models are complementary and refer to health behaviors rather than health outcomes (obesity). Moreover, they imply, without explicitly mentioning, that deprived or poor neighborhoods are structurally and functionally disadvantaged.

Indirect-effect models, such as the relationship model or the buffering model, try to capture the mediating or moderating roles of mostly family influences. In other words, they focus on indirect mechanisms through which neighborhood characteristics influence the health of children or adolescents [16, 18]. The relationship model assumes that neighborhood conditions influence the health of children or adolescents through parental (or peer) behavior, which means that neighborhood characteristics are mediated by parents or friends. For example, poverty, violence, and a lack of social support in the neighborhood may increase parental stress, disrupt family functioning, and lead to negative health outcomes in children [16, 18]. The buffering model suggests that social support (from family or friends) protects children from negative neighborhood conditions. In other words, adverse neighborhood conditions are moderated by social support that contributes to the resilience of children [16, 19].

Indirect-effect models follow a rather social ecological approach. The social ecological theory is a complex framework that emphasizes the nested (and therefore interdependent) arrangement of family, school, neighborhood, and community contexts [4]. The questions that arise are whether and how this profoundly complex framework can be empirically investigated. Although conceptual and empirical work on the relation between neighborhood characteristics and health in children and adolescents has advanced in recent decades, we are still not able to capture the complexity of how neighborhoods influence health. Changes over time, residential self-selection [20], dynamic-agent models [21], and mobility are some aspects that are seen as valuable for further theoretical and empirical research.

Implications for Research and Practice

As we have shown in our short overview, there is evidence that neighborhood characteristics contribute to unhealthy weight gain in children and adolescents. The results are impressive, but we have to be careful about generalizing because there is no 'universal 'area effect on health' [but] some area effects on some health outcomes, in some population groups, and in some types of areas' [10]. In other words, some area characteristics matter for some people in some places – but not for others. As outlined above, there are methodological and empirical discrepancies that can be traced back to a lack of use of existing theoretical frameworks, which leads to an apparently arbitrary choice of neighborhood variables without explicitly mentioning the expected influences and mechanisms [22]. Further research should try to overcome the gap between theory and empiricism by more consciously drawing on existing evidence and theory. On the one hand, researchers should employ validated, comprehensive, and at least widely used instruments and definitions to measure neighborhood characteristics in order to contribute to the evidence on the environmental influences on childhood obesity. On the other hand, innovative methodological approaches that are conducive to theoretical progress are needed.

Nevertheless, taking environmental characteristics into account is necessary for explaining inequalities in the prevalence of obesity [1]. From a public health perspective, even smaller effects at the population level are important because a great number of individuals can benefit. Moreover, the lack of effectiveness and sustainability of individual behavior-oriented interventions on lifestyle and health changes underlines the potential of environmental influences [23]. As Swerissen stated, 'interventions that isolate individual action from its social context are unlikely to produce sustainable health gains in the absence of change to the organizational, community and institutional conditions that make up the social context' [24]. Community-based interventions and community-based participatory research are promising strategies for sustainable health changes because they are aimed at producing environmental changes in a specific community by actively involving the residents [23]. Regarding obesity prevention and intervention, community-based interventions can lead to improvements in the physical environment (e.g. increases in the amount of green space and number of physical activity facilities that are easily accessible and appropriate for the target group) but also to changes in the social environment (by empowering residents, changing social norms, and increasing social capital). Finally, changing environmental characteristics might lead to a reduction in health inequalities.

References

1 Law C, Power C, Graham H, Merrick D: Obesity and health inequalities. Obes Rev 2007;8:19–22.

2 Diez Roux AV, Mair C: Neighborhoods and health. Ann N Y Acad Sci 2010;1186:125–145.

3 Carter MA, Dubois L: Neighbourhoods and child adiposity: a critical appraisal of the literature. Health Place 2010;16:616–628.

4 Earls F, Carlson M: The social ecology of child health and well-being. Annu Rev Publ Health 2001;22:143–166.

5 Cummins S, Curtis S, Diez-Roux AV, Macintyre S: Understanding and representing 'place' in health research: a relational approach. Soc Sci Med 2007;65: 1825–1838.

6 Swinburn B, Egger G, Raza F: Dissecting obesogenic environments: the development and application of a framework for identifying and prioritizing environmental interventions for obesity. Prev Med 1999;29: 563–570.

7 Dunton GF, Kaplan J, Wolch J, Jerrett M, Reynolds KD: Physical environmental correlates of childhood obesity: a systematic review. Obes Rev 2009;10:393–402.

8 El-Sayed AM, Scarborough P, Galea S: Socioeconomic inequalities in childhood obesity in the United Kingdom: a systematic review of the literature. Obes Facts 2012;5:671–692.

9 Shrewsbury V, Wardle J: Socioeconomic status and adiposity in childhood: a systematic review of cross-sectional studies 1990–2005. Obesity 2008;16:275–284.

10 Macintyre S, Ellaway A, Cummins S: Place effects on health: how can we conceptualise, operationalise and measure them? Soc Sci Med 2002;55:125–139.

11 Spence JC, Cutumisu N, Edwards J, Evans J: Influence of neighbourhood design and access to facilities on overweight among preschool children. Int J Pediatr Obes 2008;3:109–116.

12 Veitch J, van Stralen MM, Chinapaw MJM, Velde SJT, Crawford D, Salmon J, et al: The neighborhood social environment and body mass index among youth: a mediation analysis. Int J Behav Nutr Phy 2012;9:1–9.

13 Macintyre S: What are spatial effects and how can we measure them?; in Dale A (ed): Exploiting National Survey and Census Data: The Role of Locality and Spatial Effects. Manchester, CCSR, Faculty of Economic and Social Studies, University of Manchester, 1997, pp 1–17.

14 Bernard P, Charafeddine R, Frohlich KL, Daniel M, Kestens Y, Potvin L: Health inequalities and place: a theoretical conception of neighbourhood. Soc Sci Med 2007;65:1839–1852.

15 Jencks C, Mayer SE: The social consequences of growing up in a poor neighborhood; in Lynn LE, McGeary MGH (eds): Inner-City Poverty in the United States. Washington, DC, National Academy Press, 1990, pp 111–185.

16 Fan Y, Chen Q: Family functioning as a mediator between neighborhood conditions and children's health: evidence from a national survey in the United States. Soc Sci Med 2012;74:1939–1947.

17 Ellen IG, Mijanovich T, Dillman K: Neighborhood effects on health: exploring the links and assessing the evidence. J Urban Affairs 2001;23:391–408.

18 Leventhal T, Brooks-Gunn J: The neighborhoods they live in: The effects of neighborhood residence on child and adolescent outcomes. Psychol Bull 2000;126:309–337.

19 Cohen S, Wills TA: Stress, social support, and the buffering hypothesis. Psychol Bull 1985;98:310–357.

20 Boone-Heinonen J, Gordon-Larsen P, Guilkey DK, Jacobs DR Jr, Popkin BM: Environment and physical activity dynamics: the role of residential self-selection. Psychol Sport Exerc 2011;12:54–60.

21 Auchincloss AH, Diez Roux AV: A new tool for epidemiology: the usefulness of dynamic-agent models in understanding place effects on health. Am J Epidemiol 2008;168:1–8.

22 Mitchell R, Gleave S, Bartley M, Wiggins D, Joshi H: Do attitude and area influence health? A multilevel approach to health inequalities. Health Place 2000;6: 67–79.

23 Navarro V: What we mean by social determinants of health. Glob Health Promot 2009;16:5–16.

24 Swerissen H: The sustainability of health promotion interventions for different levels of social organization. Health Promot Int 2004;19:123–130.

25 Chen E, Paterson LQ: Neighborhood, family, and subjective socioeconomic status: how do they relate to adolescent health? Health Psychol 2006;25:704–714.

26 Janssen I, Boyce WF, Simpson K, Pickett W: Influence of individual- and area-level measures of socioeconomic status on obesity, unhealthy eating, and physical inactivity in Canadian adolescents. Am J Clin Nutr 2006;83:139–145.

27 Koller D, Mielck A: Regional and social differences concerning overweight, participation in health check-ups and vaccination. Analysis of data from a whole birth cohort of 6-year old children in a prosperous German city. BMC Public Health 2009;9:43.

28 Oliver LN, Hayes MV: Effects of neighbourhood income on reported body mass index: an eight year longitudinal study of Canadian children. BMC Public Health 2008;8:16.

29 Veugelers P, Sithole F, Zhang S, Muhajarine N: Neighborhood characteristics in relation to diet, physical activity and overweight of Canadian children. Int J Pediatr Obes 2008;3:152–159.
30 Grafova IB: Overweight children: assessing the contribution of the built environment. Prev Med 2008; 47:304–308.
31 Kinra S, Nelder RP, Lewendon GJ: Deprivation and childhood obesity: a cross sectional study of 20,973 children in Plymouth, United Kingdom. J Epidemiol Community Health 2000;54:456–460.
32 Oliver LN, Hayes MV: Neighbourhood socio-economic status and the prevalence of overweight Canadian children and youth. Can J Public Health 2005;96:415–420.
33 Cecil JE, Watt P, Murrie ISL, Wrieden W, Wallis DJ, Hetherington MM, et al: Childhood obesity and socioeconomic status: a novel role for height growth limitation. Int J Obes 2005;29:1199–1203.
34 Rutter H: Data briefing. Child obesity worst in deprived areas. Health Serv J 2008:21.
35 Emerson E: Overweight and obesity in 3- and 5-year-old children with and without developmental delay. Public Health 2009;123:130–133.
36 Armstrong J, Dorosty AR, Reilly JJ, Emmett PM: Coexistence of social inequalities in undernutrition and obesity in preschool children: population based cross sectional study. Arch Dis Child 2003;88:671–675.
37 Wardle J, Brodersen NH, Cole TJ, Jarvis MJ, Boniface DR: Development of adiposity in adolescence: five year longitudinal study of an ethnically and socioeconomically diverse sample of young people in Britain. BMJ 2006;332:1130–1135.
38 Jansen W, Hazebroek-Kampschreur AA: Differences in height and weight between children living in neighbourhoods of different socioeconomic status. Acta Paediatr 1997;86:224–225.
39 Scott MM, Cohen DA, Evenson KR, Elder J, Catellier D, Ashwood JS, et al: Weekend schoolyard accessibility, physical activity, and obesity: the Trial of Activity in Adolescent Girls (TAAG) study. Prev Med 2007;44:398–403.
40 Sweeting H, West P, Young R: Obesity among Scottish 15 year olds 1987–2006: prevalence and associations with socio-economic status, well-being and worries about weight. BMC Public Health 2008;8:404.
41 Wardle J, Jarvis MJ, Steggles N, Sutton S, Williamson S, Farrimond H, et al: Socioeconomic disparities in cancer-risk behaviors in adolescence: baseline results from the Health and Behaviour in Teenagers Study (HABITS). Prev Med 2003;36:721–730.
42 Booth ML, Macaskill P, Lazarus R, Baur LA: Sociodemographic distribution of measures of body fatness among children and adolescents in New South Wales, Australia. Int J Obes Relat Metab Disord 1999;23:456–462.
43 Wright CM, Parker L: Forty years on: the effect of deprivation on growth in two Newcastle birth cohorts. Int J Epidemiol 2004;33:147–152.
44 Cohen DA, Finch BK, Bower A, Sastry N: Collective efficacy and obesity: the potential influence of social factors on health. Soc Sci Med 2006;62:769–778.
45 Brunt H, Lester N, Davies G, Williams R: Childhood overweight and obesity: is the gap closing the wrong way? J Public Health (Oxf) 2008;30:145–152.
46 Dummer TJ, Gibbon MA, Hackett AF, Stratton G, Taylor SR: Is overweight and obesity in 9–10-year-old children in Liverpool related to deprivation and/or electoral ward when based on school attended? Public Health Nutr 2005;8:636–641.
47 Burke V, Beilin LJ, Dunbar D, Kevan M: Associations between blood pressure and overweight defined by new standards for body mass index in childhood. Prev Med 2004;38:558–564.
48 Cowell JM, Warren JS, Montgomery AC: Cardiovascular risk prevalence among diverse school-age children: implications for schools. J Sch Nurs 1999;15:8–12.
49 Bell JF, Wilson JS, Liu GC: Neighborhood greenness and 2-year changes in body mass index of children and youth. Am J Prev Med 2008;35:547–553.
50 Liu GC, Wilson JS, Qi R, Ying J: Green neighborhoods, food retail and childhood overweight: differences by population density. Am J Health Promot 2007;21:317–325.
51 Norman GJ, Nutter S, Ryan S, Sallis J, Calfas K, Patrick K: Community design and access to recreational facilities as correlates of adolescent physical activity and body-mass index. J Phys Act Health 2006;3: S118–S128.
52 Kligerman M, Sallis JF, Ryan S, Frank LD, Nader PR: Association of neighborhood design and recreation environment variables with physical activity and body mass index in adolescents. Am J Health Promot 2007;21:274–277.
53 Gordon-Larsen P, Nelson MC, Page P, Popkin BM: Inequality in the built environment underlies key health disparities in physical activity and obesity. Pediatr 2006;117:417–424.
54 Evenson KR, Scott MM, Cohen DA, Voorhees CC: Girls' perception of neighborhood factors on physical activity, sedentary behavior, and BMI. Obesity (Silver Spring) 2007;15:430–445.
55 Burdette HL, Whitaker RC: Neighborhood playgrounds, fast food restaurants, and crime: relationships to overweight in low-income preschool children. Prev Med 2004;38:57–63.

56 Timperio A, Salmon J, Telford A, Crawford D: Perceptions of local neighbourhood environments and their relationship to childhood overweight and obesity. Int J Obes (Lond) 2005;29:170–175.
57 Merchant AT, Dehghan M, Behnke-Cook D, Anand SS: Diet, physical activity, and adiposity in children in poor and rich neighbourhoods: a cross-sectional comparison. Nutr J 2007;6:1.
58 McKay CM, Bell-Ellison BA, Wallace K, Ferron JM: A multilevel study of the associations between economic and social context, stage of adolescence, and physical activity and body mass index. Pediatr 2007; 119(suppl 1):S84–S91.
59 Burdette HL, Whitaker RC: A national study of neighborhood safety, outdoor play, television viewing, and obesity in preschool children. Pediatr 2005; 116:657–662.
60 Lumeng JC, Appugliese D, Cabral HJ, Bradley RH, Zuckerman B: Neighborhood safety and overweight status in children. Arch Pediatr Adolesc Med 2006; 160:25–31.
61 O'Brien M, Nader PR, Houts RM, Bradley R, Friedman SL, Belsky J, et al: The ecology of childhood overweight: a 12-year longitudinal analysis. Int J Obes (Lond) 2007;31:1469–1478.

Dipl. Soz.arb./Soz.päd. Ulrike Igel
Faculty of Architecture and Social Sciences
Leipzig University of Applied Sciences (HTWK Leipzig)
POB 301166
DE–04251 Leipzig (Germany)
E-Mail ulrike.igel@htwk-leipzig.de

Kiess W, Wabitsch M, Maffeis C, Sharma AM (eds): Metabolic Syndrome and Obesity in Childhood and Adolescence.
Pediatr Adolesc Med. Basel, Karger, 2015, vol 19, pp 137–147 (DOI: 10.1159/000368125)

Metabolic Syndrome and the 'Western Diet': Science and Politics

Robert H. Lustig[a, b]

[a]Division of Pediatric Endocrinology, Department of Pediatrics, UCSF Benioff Children's Hospital and the
[b]Philip R. Lee Institute for Health Policy Studies, University of California, San Francisco, Calif., USA

Abstract

Metabolic syndrome comprises a set of chronic diseases (hypertension, diabetes, dyslipidemia, and cardiovascular disease) that tend to cluster together. Although obesity is commonly thought to be the antecedent of metabolic syndrome, this syndrome also occurs in lean individuals, suggesting that obesity is a marker of metabolic syndrome rather than a cause. The cellular mechanisms of metabolic syndrome include mitochondrial overload, *de novo* lipogenesis, hepatic insulin resistance and hyperinsulinemia, reactive oxygen species formation, endoplasmic reticulum stress, and the unfolded protein response. Specific alterations of the Western Diet uniquely drive this process and are unrelated to calories. These alterations include too little fiber, omega-3 fatty acids, and micronutrients, and too many omega-6 fatty acids, *trans*-fats, branched-chain amino acids, ethanol, and fructose. The food industry invokes personal responsibility while denying any corporate responsibility and citing scientific, policy, and social arguments. However, their responses obfuscate the scientific truth in order to obviate their culpability.

Introduction

'Metabolic syndrome' is routinely defined by physicians and medical societies as a constellation of chronic diseases that encompass obesity, type 2 diabetes, hypertension, dyslipidemia, and cardiovascular disease. Since the inception of this term, we have learned about other diseases that also co-migrate with metabolic syndrome, including polycystic ovarian syndrome and nonalcoholic fatty liver disease. Preliminary data also argue that cancer and dementia are ancillary diseases within the new scope of the term 'metabolic syndrome'. All of these diseases are chronic metabolic diseases that have increased in prevalence in adults since 1980, when dietary guidelines across the world changed. Worse yet, all of these diseases were unheard of in children before 1980, but now, 13% of normal-weight children and 38% of obese children harbor these same chronic metabolic diseases. Furthermore, obesity and type 2 diabetes now exist side-by-side in developing nations where hunger and undernutrition still manifest. When examining the global pattern of spread, this looks much more like an exposure than a behavior.

Metabolic Syndrome

Six separate medical societies (World Health Organization 1998, European Group for the Study of Insulin Resistance 1998, National Cholesterol Education Program/Adult Treatment Panel III 2001, American Association of Clinical Endocrinologists 2003, International Diabetes Federation 2005, and American Heart Association 2005) have defined metabolic syndrome differently, based on cutoffs for body mass index, waist circumference, blood pressure, triglyceride (TG) levels, and blood glucose. These differences mean that at least five of the societies, and likely all six, have gotten it wrong. A pediatric writing group of the American Heart Association in 2009 did not even try to define metabolic syndrome in children [1]. The problems with the current definitions of metabolic syndrome are three-fold. First, since each of the hallmark diseases occurs in a unicameral but kurtotic distribution, rather than a bimodal distribution, it is impossible to draw appropriate cutoff points. For instance, saying that the 91st percentile for blood pressure is metabolic syndrome, while the 90th percentile is not, is begging for misclassification. Second, virtually all of the definitions utilize obesity as a defining feature, but they do not explain the syndrome of lipodystrophy (an absence of subcutaneous fat), where all fat is stored in liver and muscle, causing severe insulin resistance and diabetes [2]. In fact, metabolic syndrome can arise from too much or too little fat; in other words, it is not the fat that counts. Third, 20% of the obese population is metabolically normal; conversely, 40% of the normal-weight population has the same metabolic dysfunction as the obese. Obesity is a *marker* for metabolic dysfunction, not a *cause*. Metabolic syndrome is from an exposure, not a behavior, and anyone and everyone is at risk.

Hepatic Insulin Resistance

Many of the definitions of metabolic syndrome infer antecedent insulin resistance [3]. However, not all tissues are equally resistant to insulin. In general, marked insulin resistance results in global metabolic dysfunction, such as leprechaunism or Rabson-Mendenhall syndrome, with virtually no fat accumulation. Thus, insulin resistance must affect different tissues and different signal transduction pathways within the same tissue differently and quantitatively. Of the eight tissue-specific insulin receptor knockout mice developed at the Joslin Diabetes Center, only the liver insulin receptor knockout and the brain insulin receptor knockout manifest obesity [4].

The liver is the primary target of insulin action. Insulin binds to the hepatic insulin receptor and elicits two key metabolic pathways. First, insulin stimulates the phosphorylation of forkhead protein O1 (FoxO1), which excludes FoxO1 from the nucleus

[5], thus diminishing the expression of genes required for gluconeogenesis, reducing hepatic glucose output, and maintaining euglycemia. Second, insulin activates sterol regulatory element-binding protein (SREBP)-1c, which in turn increases the transcription of genes required for fatty acid and TG biosynthesis (ATP-citrate lyase, acetyl-coenzyme A carboxylase, and fatty acid synthase), which collectively constitute the process of *de novo* lipogenesis (DNL). TGs synthesized in the liver by DNL have two fates. TGs can be packaged with apoliprotein B into very low-density lipoproteins for export to the periphery or for storage or utilization and therefore can drive cardiovascular disease and/or obesity. Alternatively, TGs can precipitate in the liver without being exported, thus promoting hepatic steatosis, which promotes hepatic insulin resistance, generates hyperinsulinemia, and increases the risk for diabetes [6].

Patients with metabolic syndrome typically have 'selective' or 'dissociated' hepatic insulin resistance; that is, they have reduced phosphorylation of FoxO1 (leading to hyperglycemia) but enhanced hepatic DNL (mediated by the SREBP-1c pathway) [7], leading to hypertriglyceridemia, ectopic lipid deposition, and fatty liver disease. If there is only one insulin receptor, how can hepatic insulin resistance lead to the diminution of one liver pathway yet the accentuation of the other?

Ectopic Lipid Partitioning

Ectopic lipid partitioning refers to the distribution of body fat in various organs such as muscle and liver instead of subcutaneously. Associations between visceral adiposity, insulin resistance, and co-morbidities have been demonstrated across most age groups and ethnicities. Studies performed in obese adolescents highlight the fact that the ratio of visceral to subcutaneous fat rather than their absolute quantity may determine their metabolic impact. Indeed, obese adolescents with a high ratio, who are not necessarily more obese than others, demonstrate a markedly adverse metabolic phenotype of severe insulin resistance and alterations in glucose and lipid metabolism. Moreover, intrahepatic fat, while being strongly associated with high levels of visceral fat, is independently associated with the insulin-resistance state in obese adolescents and is independent of all other fat depots [8]. Alternatively, the lipid content of insulin responsive tissues, such as liver and/or muscle, is increased in obesity and in type 2 diabetes mellitus and is a strong predictor of insulin resistance [6]. Furthermore, lipid deposition in hepatocytes to produce intrahepatocellular lipid is highly predictive of insulin resistance, even more so than visceral fat [9]. The accumulation of lipids, in particular diacyl glycerol, activates the hepatic inflammatory cascade by inducing c-jun N-terminal kinase (JNK-1), which causes serine rather than tyrosine phosphorylation of IRS-1, leading to inhibition of hepatic insulin signaling.

One hypothesis suggests that once the subcutaneous fat depot reaches its storage capacity and begins to shunt lipid to ectopic tissues (such as liver and muscle), peripheral insulin resistance ensues. Another hypothesis is that the liver accumulates fat produced by DNL and reduces fat β-oxidation in response to dietary factors, such as components of fast food (see below).

Reactive Oxygen Species, Endoplasmic Reticulum Stress, and the Unfolded Protein Response

The 'Free Radical Theory' holds that an imbalance between reactive oxygen species (ROS) generation and antioxidant defenses is a major factor in DNA and cellular damage leading to metabolic syndrome. Excessive nutrient processing by mitochondria can result in uncoupling of oxidative phosphorylation and in increased generation of ROS, which, in turn, alters mitochondrial function and further increases ROS generation. ROS that are not quenched by antioxidants in peroxisomes find their way to the adjacent endoplasmic reticulum (ER), where they alter the redox environment that is crucial for proper protein folding. Accumulation of ROS and misfolded proteins within the ER activates the unfolded protein response (UPR), which is designed to decrease protein synthesis in order to allow the clearance of misfolded proteins. ER stress in the liver is a specific mechanism of hepatic injury in nonalcoholic fatty liver disease [10], and ER stress in the pancreas reduces β-cell numbers and promotes type 2 diabetes [11].

The Western Diet

While overnutrition of total calories ingested has routinely been implicated in the pathogenesis of obesity, it does not explain why some obese people develop metabolic syndrome and others do not or why normal-weight people develop metabolic syndrome. Furthermore, obesity prevalence is increasing worldwide by 1% per year, while diabetes prevalence is increasing by 4% per year. Rather, the quality of the calories taken in likely plays a major role in the pathogenesis of the metabolic syndrome through hepatic mitochondrial overload, hepatic insulin resistance, fatty liver disease and ROS formation. In fact, three nutrient deficiencies and five nutrient excesses within the Western Diet have been specifically implicated in the pathogenesis of metabolic syndrome and are unrelated to obesity.

Too Little Fiber

When fiber (soluble and insoluble) is consumed with a meal, it forms a gelatinous barrier between the food and the intestinal wall, which delays the intestine's ability to absorb glucose, fructose, and fat. By slowing glucose absorption, the rise in blood glucose is attenuated, which limits the peak glucose level, resulting in an attenuated insulin response. In the Insulin Resistance and Atherosclerosis Study, dietary analysis demonstrated that the only food item that correlated with insulin sensitivity was fiber. However, other studies showed that improvement in insulin sensitivity was conferred by a dose of insoluble fiber. When patients with type 2 diabetes ate a high-fiber diet, their blood sugar levels were cut by one-third, which reduced the total insulin load of the body [12].

Too Few Omega-3 Fatty Acids

Omega-3 fatty acids, which are found in wild fish and flax, serve as precursors to docahexaenoic acid and eicosopentanoic acid and are notably anti-inflammatory. Conversely omega-6 fatty acids, which are found in seed oils, are precursors of arachidonic acid and are notably pro-inflammatory. Nutritionists suggest that our ratio of omega-6 to omega-3 fatty acids should be approximately 1:1. Currently, our ratio is about 25:1, which sets up a pro-inflammatory state that drives ROS formation and cell damage.

Too Few Micronutrients

Antioxidants are required to help quench ROS to prevent ER stress and cellular damage. Antioxidants come in many shapes and sizes, many of which have been considered treatments for metabolic syndrome [13]. The antioxidants vitamins C and E protect against lipid peroxidation, although neither has been shown to directly improve vascular function or insulin resistance. Many epidemiologic studies demonstrate correlations between low blood levels of antioxidants such as vitamin C and beta-carotene and the prevalence of metabolic syndrome. However, it is not yet clear whether these micronutrient deficiencies are the true cause of disease or if they are just markers of an extremely poor diet. When the diet is altered to deliver more of these compounds, metabolic syndrome improves. However, when antioxidants are given as dietary supplements, they usually fail miserably. This difference in effects could very well be due to the beneficial effects of eating unprocessed foods, in which fiber is high and the antioxidants are a bonus.

Too Many Trans-Fats

Trans-fats cannot be completely metabolized by mitochondria due to the *trans*-double bond, and they line arteries and the liver and generate increased levels of ROS species. *Trans*-fats have long been assumed to contribute to chronic metabolic disease, especially atherosclerosis (hardening of the arteries). Of note, on November 7, 2013, the U.S. Food and Drug Administration declared that *trans*-fats are not 'generally recognized as safe', ensuring their eventual disappearance from the American food supply.

Too Many Branched-Chain Amino Acids

The branched-chain amino acids (BCAAs) valine, leucine, and isoleucine are essential amino acids that account for >20% of the amino acids in the typical 'Western Diet'. In the anabolic (childhood growth and puberty, body building) state, these amino acids are required for new protein biosynthesis, especially in muscle. However, when provided in excess beyond anabolic requirements, they are deaminated in the liver and diverted directly to the mitochondria for energy utilization [14]. BCAAs increase SREBP-1c without insulin regulation, facilitating DNL. Furthermore, BCAAs promote the serine phosphorylation of IRS-1 and impair insulin signaling. Lastly, chronic BCAA elevation impairs the transport of aromatic amino acids into the brain, and the reduced production of serotonin (derived from tryptophan) and catecholamines (derived from phenylalanine and tyrosine) may drive hunger [14]. The 'BCAA overload' hypothesis suggests that BCAAs may make an independent contribution to the development of hepatic insulin resistance.

Too Much Ethanol

Although adult epidemiological studies associate light to moderate ethanol consumption with improved insulin sensitivity and wine consumption with reduced cardiovascular risk, other cross-sectional and prospective studies implicate a dose-dependent effect of alcohol on metabolic syndrome and suggest that chronic consumption of large amounts of ethanol worsen insulin sensitivity. Ethanol bypasses glycolysis by being converted to acetaldehyde by alcohol dehydrogenase-1B, which promotes ROS formation and must also be quenched by hepatic antioxidants such as glutathione or ascorbic acid to prevent cellular damage. Acetaldehyde is then metabolized to acetic acid by the enzyme aldehyde dehydrogenase-2, which, in turn, is metabolized to form acetyl-CoA by the enzyme acyl-CoA synthetase short-chain family member 2. Excess acetyl-CoA can overload mitochondria without insulin regulation and is preferentially used for the synthesis of TG through DNL. While clearly a concern in adults, it is unlikely that ethanol contributes significantly to metabolic syndrome in children.

Too Much Fructose

The most commonly used sweetener in the U.S. diet is the disaccharide sucrose (e.g., table sugar), which contains 50% fructose and 50% glucose. However, in North America and many other countries, nondiet soft drinks are sweetened with high-fructose corn syrup (HFCS), which contains up to 55% of the monosaccharide fructose. Due to its abundance, sweetness, and low price, HFCS has become the most common sweetener used in processed foods. Average daily fructose consumption has increased by over 25% over the past 30 years, and the growing dependence on fructose (especially with the reduction in dietary fat) in the Western Diet may be fueling the obesity and type 2 diabetes epidemics. Animal and human models demonstrate that high-fructose diets lead to increased energy intake, decreased resting energy expenditure, excess fat deposition, and insulin resistance (fig. 1) [15, 16].

Only the liver has the Glut5 transporter; thus, in the fed state, the overwhelming majority of fructose metabolism occurs in the liver. Fructose is rapidly metabolized to fructose-1-phosphate (F1P) via fructokinase, an insulin-independent process that also bypasses the negative feedback regulation of phosphofructokinase in the glycolytic pathway. Thus, fructose metabolism generates lipogenic substrates (e.g., glyceraldehyde-3-phosphate and acetyl-CoA) in an unregulated fashion, and these substrates are delivered straight to the mitochondria, driving hepatic DNL, and will either be exported as TG or will possibly overwhelm the liver's lipid export capacity, leading to intrahepatic lipid deposition and hepatic steatosis. F1P also stimulates SREBP-1c via peroxisome proliferator-activated receptor-gamma co-activator (PGC)-1β [17] independently of insulin, which activates the genes involved in DNL. Additionally,

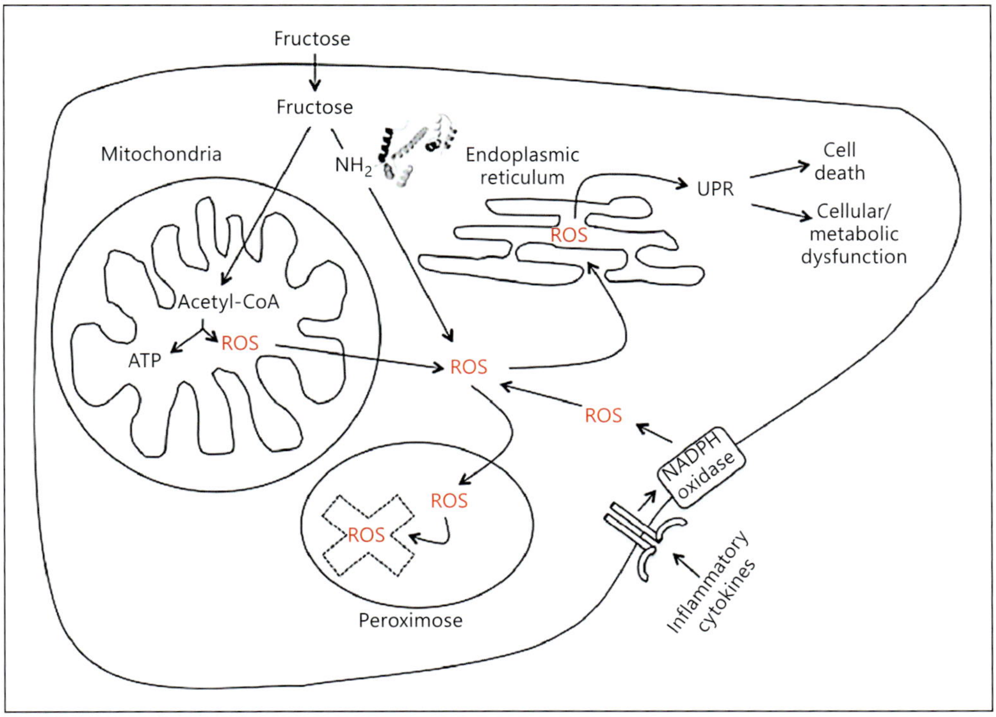

Fig. 1. Mechanisms of subcellular metabolic dysfunction, using fructose as an example. The formation of acetyl-CoA leads to lipid deposition and activation of inflammatory pathways, which serine phosphorylate IRS-1, leading to insulin resistance. Furthermore, metabolic processing in the mitochondria, the glycation of protein ε-amino groups via the Maillard reaction, and circulating inflammatory cytokines, due to their receptor-mediated activation of NADPH oxidase, all increase the intracellular levels of ROS. In the absence of sufficient peroxisomal quenching and degradation, the ROS moieties lead to endoplasmic reticulum stress, promoting the unfolded protein response and causing either cell death (apoptosis) or cellular/metabolic dysfunction, from [20]. Courtesy of the American Academy of Pediatrics. ATP = Adenosine triphosphate; CoA = coenzyme A; JNK-1 = c-jun N-terminal kinase 1; NADPH = nicotinamide adenine dinucleotide phosphate; PKCε, protein kinase C−ε; pSer-IRS-1, serine phosphorylated IRS-1; ROS, reactive oxygen species; UPR, unfolded protein response.

F1P activates dual-specificity mitogen-activated protein kinase 7 (MKK7), which subsequently stimulates JNK-1 and serine phosphorylates IRS-1, inactivating it, which leads to hepatic insulin resistance.

In addition, due to its unique stereochemistry, the ring form of fructose (a five-membered furan with axial hydroxymethyl groups) is under a great deal of ionic strain, which favors the linear form of the molecule that exposes the reactive 2-keto group, which can readily engage in the nonenzymatic fructosylation of exposed amino moieties of proteins via the Maillard reaction in the same way that the 1-aldehyde position of glucose is reactive with proteins. Each Maillard reaction generates one ROS, which must be quenched by an antioxidant at the risk of cellular damage. Thus, fructose generates excessive ROS, which can lead to cellular damage and promote ER stress and metabolic syndrome.

Two recent studies support sugar as a specific and direct causative agent of type 2 diabetes. A prospective analysis of the European Prospective Investigation into Cancer-InterAct study found that sugared beverage consumption increased risk for diabetes development by 29%, exclusive of its calories or of body mass index [18]. Our group showed that global sugar availability predicted the prevalence of diabetes during the decade 2000–2010, exclusive of total calories, calories from other foodstuffs, aging, obesity, physical activity, or income. For every 150 calories per day in excess, diabetes prevalence increased 0.1%, but if those 150 calories happened to be a can of soda, diabetes prevalence increased 11-fold, by 1.1% [19].

Dietary Quality Matters More than Dietary Quantity

Trans-fats, BCAAs, ethanol, and fructose are more alike than different. They all share three biochemical properties: (1) they are metabolized for energy primarily within the liver; (2) they are not regulated by insulin; and (3) they do not have a 'pop-off' mechanism to form glycogen for storage, rather, they go straight to the mitochondria as acetyl-CoA, which can cause mitochondrial overload, ROS generation, excessive DNL, and impaired β-oxidation, which drives hepatic insulin resistance, hepatic steatosis, ROS production, ER stress, and results in metabolic syndrome. Thus, food processing, by removing important nutrients and adding potentially toxic nutrients, specifically drives the development of metabolic syndrome, exclusive of calories or obesity [20].

The Food Industry Responds

As one might expect, the food industry denies any culpability in fomenting the pandemic of metabolic syndrome and challenges the veracity of these arguments on physical, biochemical, policy, and social grounds.

A Calorie Is a Calorie

The food industry argues that obesity obeys the first law of thermodynamics, that obesity is about energy balance, and therefore that obesity is a manifestation of two behaviors: increased intake (gluttony) and decreased expenditure (sloth), ascribing blame to the individual. However, as discussed above, obesity is not the issue; metabolic syndrome is the issue, and for metabolic syndrome, dietary quality matters more than quantity.

Animals Are Not Humans

The food industry is quick to point out that most fructose studies are done in rodents using large doses over a short period of time. A recent study in rats showed that sugar at normal levels of consumption could cause morbidity and mortality

[21]. Furthermore, studies done in primates demonstrated similar detrimental effects [15]. Lastly, human feeding studies were consistent with the analogies shown above [16].

Fructose Does Not Raise Blood Glucose

The industry argues that fructose does not raise blood glucose levels. It has a very low glycemic index, of 19 (glucose is the index at 100). The glycemic index is a measure of a food's generation of an insulin response and is used as a method for quantifying a food's potential for weight gain. Indeed, fructose alone does not raise blood glucose levels, nor does it generate an insulin response. Fructose is worse because it raises the blood fructose level, which leads to ROS formation in the liver and in arterial walls. Additionally, fructose is not found alone in nature; it is always found paired with glucose (either as sucrose or HFCS), and the glucose contribution generates quite a hefty insulin response.

Fructose Does Not Raise Hemoglobin A1c

The food industry argues that because fructose does not raise the blood glucose level, it also does not increase hemoglobin A1c levels. In the blood, fructose does not bind to the amino moiety at position 1 of hemoglobin to generate hemoglobin A1c (leading the food industry to wrongly assume that fructose is benign); rather, fructation occurs at positions 7, 66, and 127 of the hemoglobin molecule [22]. Thus, the damage from nonenzymatic fructosylation does occur, but it is not measured at position 1.

Fructose for Glucose Exchange Studies Show No Detrimental Effects

Meta-analyses of controlled isocaloric 'fructose for glucose' exchange studies demonstrate no effects of weight gain or other morbidities [23]. Perhaps one reason for this absence of effect is because crystalline fructose is incompletely absorbed, and thus its effects on glucose and HbA_{1c} may be minimal. However, fructose malabsorption can cause significant gastrointestinal distress, such as pain, bloating, and diarrhea. Furthermore, the meta-analyses where fructose was supplied in excess showed weight gain, dyslipidemia, and insulin resistance [23]. Thus, the dose determines the poison.

During fasting (glycogen-depletion) in normal-weight individuals, DNL of oral fructose occurs at a rate of less than 5% [24]. However, in obese, insulin-resistant, fed individuals consuming both fructose and glucose together, the DNL of fructose occurs at a much higher rate, approximately 30% [25]. In other words, the toxicity of fructose depends on the context.

The Ingredients Are on the Label

The food industry counters that the information is on the Nutrition Facts label in order to educate the public properly. However, this is only half true. The Nutrition Labeling and Education Act of 1990 requires the disclosure of *total sugars* on the

Nutrition Facts Label for processed food, which includes the endogenous sugar in the food itself, the lactose in the milk, and the added sucrose or HFCS. An example of industry subterfuge is yogurt. A six-ounce plain yogurt has 7 g of sugar, all lactose. However, a six-ounce pomegranate yogurt has 19 g of sugar, indicating that 12 g of sugar was added, the same as in a bowl of sweetened cereal. Furthermore, there are 56 names for sugar, most of which are unknown to the public. As the label lists ingredients by mass, a food company can use different sugars as ingredients #5, #6, #7, and #8; when you do the math, they can add up to #1.

Individuals Are Personally Responsible for Their Dietary Choices

Personal responsibility requires knowledge, access, and affordability. Clearly, people are being denied the knowledge of what goes into their food. Furthermore, of the 600,000 food items in the American grocery store, 80% contain sugar added by the food industry for its own purposes [26]. Lower-socioecomic-status individuals rarely have access to 'real food', and public health nutrition programs provide processed rather than real food. Thus, many people are not responsible for their dietary choices.

Conclusions

Metabolic syndrome overlaps with obesity, but it is a distinct entity, as it occurs in normal-weight individuals as well, and children suffer from metabolic syndrome at a rate that is higher than their degree of obesity. The food environment plays a major role; in particular, the Western Diet, which is now the Industrial Global Diet, as it has been adopted around the world for its convenience, taste, shelf-life, and expense. Fast food and highly processed food is now prevalent and plentiful around the globe due to international trade policies. In developing countries, soda costs less than potable water or milk. Specific components in the Western Diet deliver energy directly to the mitochondria, resulting in overload, DNL, hepatic insulin resistance, ROS formation, and ER stress, which result in cellular dysfunction and death. The food industry's counterarguments are without foundation, but until the composition of processed food is altered, do not expect the diseases of metabolic syndrome to improve or abate.

References

1 Steinberger J, Daniels SR, Eckel RH, et al: Progress and challenges in metabolic syndrome in children and adolescents: a scientific statement from the American Heart Association Atherosclerosis, Hypertension, and Obesity in the Young Committee of the Council on Cardiovascular Disease in the Young; Council on Cardiovascular Nursing; and Council on Nutrition, Physical Activity, and Metabolism. Circulation 2009; 119:628–647.

2 Garg A: Acquired and inherited lipodystrophies. N Engl J Med 2004;350:1220–1234.

3 Reaven G: Role of insulin resistance in human disease (syndrome X): an expanded definition. Annu Rev Med 1993;44:121–131.

4 Haas JT, Biddinger SB: Dissecting the role of insulin resistance in the metabolic syndrome. Curr Opin Lipidol 2009;20:206–210.

5 Naïmi M, Gautier N, Chaussade C, Valverde AM, Accili D, Van Obberghen E: Nuclear forkhead box O1 controls and integrates key signaling pathways in hepatocytes. Endocrinol 2007;148:2424–2434.
6 Sung KC, Kim SH: Interrelationship between fatty liver and insulin resistance in the development of type 2 diabetes. J Clin Endocrinol Metab 2011;96:1093–1097.
7 Brown MS, Goldstein JL: Selective versus total insulin resistance: a pathogenic paradox. Cell Metab 2008;7:95–96.
8 D'Adamo E, Cali AM, Weiss R, et al: Central role of fatty liver in the pathogenesis of insulin resistance in obese adolescents. Diab Care 2010;33:1817–1822.
9 Fabbrini E, Magkos F, Mohammed BS, et al: Intrahepatic fat, not visceral fat, is linked with metabolic complications of obesity. Proc Natl Acad Sci 2009; 106:15430–15435.
10 Mollica MP, Lionetti L, Putti R, Cavaliere G, Gaita M, Barletta A: From chronic overfeeding to hepatic injury: role of endoplasmic reticulum stress and inflammation. Nutr Metab Cardiovasc Dis 2011;21:222–230.
11 Hummasti S, Hotamisligil GS: Endoplasmic reticulum stress and inflammation in obesity and diabetes. Circ Res 2010;107:579–591.
12 Weickert MO, Pfeiffer AFH: Metabolic effects of dietary fiber consumption and prevention of diabetes. J Nutr 2008;138:439–442.
13 Davì G, Santilli F, Patrono C: Nutraceuticals in diabetes and metabolic syndrome. Cardiovasc Ther 2010;28:216–226.
14 Newgard CB, An J, Bain JR, et al: A branched-chain amino acid-related metabolic signature that differentiates obese and lean humans and contributes to insulin resistance. Cell Metab 2009;9:311–326.
15 Bremer AA, Stanhope KL, Graham JL, et al: Fructose-fed rhesus monkeys: a nonhuman primate model of insulin resistance, metabolic syndrome, and type 2 diabetes. Clin Transl Sci 2011;4:243–252.
16 Stanhope KL, Schwarz JM, Keim NL, et al: Consuming fructose-, not glucose-sweetened beverages increases visceral adiposity and lipids and decreases insulin sensitivity in overweight/obese humans. J Clin Invest 2009;119:1322–1334.
17 Nagai Y, Yonemitsu S, Erion DM, et al: The role of peroxisome proliferator-activated receptor gamma coactivator-1 beta in the pathogenesis of fructose-induced insulin resistance. Cell Metab 2009;9:252–264.
18 EPIC-Interact Consortium: Consumption of sweet beverages and type 2 diabetes incidence in European adults: results from EPIC-InterAct. Diabetologia 2013;56:1520–1530.
19 Basu S, Yoffe P, Hills N, Lustig RH: The relationship of sugar to population-level diabetes prevalence: an econometric analysis of repeated cross-sectional data. PLoS One 2013;8:e57873.
20 Bremer AA, Mietus-Snyder ML, Lustig RH: Toward a unifying hypothesis of metabolic syndrome. Pediatrics 2012;129:557–570.
21 Ruff JS, Suchy AK, Hugentobler SA, et al: Human-relevant levels of added sugar consumption increase female mortality and lower male fitness in mice. Nat Commun 2013;4:2245.
22 Bose T, Chakraborti AS: Fructose-induced structural and functional modifications of hemoglobin: implication for oxidative stress in diabetes mellitus. Biochim Biophys Acta 2008;1780:800–808.
23 Sievenpiper JL, de Souza RJ, Mirrahimi A, et al: Effect of fructose on body weight in controlled feeding trials: a systematic review and meta-analysis. Ann Int Med 2012;156:291–304.
24 Parks EJ, Krauss RM, Christiansen MP, Neese RA, Hellerstein MK: Effects of a low-fat, high-carbohydrate diet on VLDL-triglyceride assembly, production, and clearance. J Clin Invest 1999;104:1087–1096.
25 Hudgins LC, Parker TS, Levine DM, Hellerstein MK: A dual sugar challenge test for lipogenic sensitivity to dietary fructose. J Clin Endocrinol Metab 2011;96: 861–868.
26 Ng SW, Slining MM, Popkin BM: Use of caloric and noncaloric sweeteners in US consumer packaged foods, 2005–2009. J Acad Nutr Diet 2012;112:1828–1834.

Robert H. Lustig, MD, MSL
Division of Pediatric Endocrinology
Department of Pediatrics, Box 0434
UCSF Benioff Children's Hospital
550 16th Street, 4th Floor
San Francisco, CA 94158–0434 (USA)
E-Mail rlustig@peds.ucsf.edu

Kiess W, Wabitsch M, Maffeis C, Sharma AM (eds): Metabolic Syndrome and Obesity in Childhood and Adolescence.
Pediatr Adolesc Med. Basel, Karger, 2015, vol 19, pp 148–159 (DOI: 10.1159/000368126)

An Economic Perspective on Childhood Obesity

Christina M. Teuner • Jürgen John • Silke B. Wolfenstetter • Rolf Holle

Helmholtz Zentrum München, German Research Center for Environmental Health, Institute of Health Economics and Health Care Management, Munich, Germany

Abstract

This review provides an overview on the latest literature on the costs of childhood and adolescent obesity and on the cost-effectiveness of interventions to prevent or manage this problem. Findings on the economic burden of childhood obesity are inconclusive, and the majority of the identified studies found excess healthcare costs for obese compared with normal-weight children by analysing different cost components and age groups. However, there are several limitations to these studies, e.g. short study periods and a strong focus on healthcare costs, disregarding other components of the economic burden of childhood obesity. Economic evaluation studies of childhood and adolescent obesity programmes indicate that cost-effective, in some cases even cost-saving, preventive and management interventions do exist. However, because of the strong variation in methodological aspects, it is difficult to compare preventive and treatment approaches in terms of their cost-effectiveness. To design effective public policies, a better understanding of these economic aspects of childhood and adolescent obesity is necessary. This understanding, however, depends on the collection of additional longitudinal data. Economic evaluation of childhood obesity interventions poses various methodological challenges that should be addressed in further research in order to support decision making.

Background

Even though evidence from several countries suggests that the rise in the prevalence of childhood obesity has slowed down (e.g. [1]), the worldwide high prevalence of childhood obesity is still alarming. This is mainly because of its serious effects on health, but there are also important economic aspects to be considered. On the one hand, there are underlying economic causes of obesity, such as technological developments and changes in the prices of goods and commodities. On the other hand, there are serious economic consequences, such as lower skill attainment and academic outcomes, worse labour market outcomes and an increasing economic burden in terms of healthcare costs and productivity losses [2]. Considering the already existing trend of increasing medical expenditure and its enhancement by ageing populations, from a policy perspective, there are two topics of special interest: the cost burden to the healthcare system that is associated with childhood obesity and the search for cost-effective intervention programmes to prevent and/or manage childhood obesity. Therefore, this chapter aims to summarise the current economic literature to provide a short update of earlier reviews of studies on these two aspects of childhood and adolescent obesity [3, 4] and to offer further research perspectives. First, this chapter focuses on the economic burden of childhood and adolescent obesity, and second, it focuses on the cost-effectiveness of programmes for preventing or treating childhood obesity.

Economic Burden of Childhood Obesity

Cost-of-Illness Studies: Methodological Aspects

When comparing different cost-of-illness studies, several methodological aspects have to be considered, as they can lead to considerable differences in the resulting cost estimates [5]. One of the most important aspects of cost-of-illness studies is the choice of the perspective (e.g. societal, health insurance, hospital, or patient perspective), as it defines which cost components are to be included in the particular analysis. The societal perspective is often preferred and recommended because all types of resources that are consumed due to illness are considered, including direct (medical and non-medical) as well as indirect costs (mostly production losses caused by illness). However, until now, almost all cost analyses of childhood obesity have focused exclusively on its direct medical costs.

Depending on what kind of epidemiological data are used, prevalence- and incidence-based cost-of-illness analyses may be distinguished. While prevalence-based studies cross-sectionally measure the incurred total costs within a defined period of time (usually 1 year), the incidence-based method longitudinally measures the economic burden from the onset of the disease to healing or death and is mostly based on simulation techniques.

In a top-down approach, highly aggregated data, such as official and administrative statistics of health expenditures that are classified according to diagnosis groups (e.g. based on International Classification of Diseases (ICD) 10 codes), are used. Usually, the costs of preventing or treating obesity itself as well as the costs of important obesity-related comorbidities, such as diabetes mellitus type 2 or cardiovascular diseases, according to their obesity-attributable fraction, are included. However, top-down cost figures often are rather imprecise, above all due to a lack of epidemiological as well as diagnosis-related expenditure data. Alternatively, in a bottom-up approach, primary data, such as health claims data, patient records, or survey data, are analysed. Since identification of obesity-related health care is often difficult, the excess-cost method, where patient-level cost data of individuals with and without the disease are compared while adjusting for several confounding variables using regression and/or matching techniques, is used. The resulting cost differences are considered to reflect the costs attributable to obesity and its comorbidities.

In health surveys, the utilisation of healthcare services is first assessed by a structured interview or self-administered questionnaire, and then the average prices (so-called 'unit costs') are used to calculate costs. More precise cost estimates are available in health claims data; however, these data usually do not contain valid information on clinical data such as body mass index (BMI), and obesity-related ICD diagnoses may be missing. The comparison of cost estimates from different studies is further complicated by differences in countries and year of reference, although economic approaches to achieve comparability do exist.

Cost-of-Illness Studies: Results of Recent Studies

Obesity during childhood can lead to a number of short-term adverse health outcomes that may be associated with increased healthcare utilisation and costs in cross-sectional studies. Two recent reviews found 21 cost-of-illness studies on childhood obesity that were published between 2006 and 2011 [3, 4]. These will be summarised below, with the addition of the latest literature through 2013.

With the exception of one early German study that estimated high incremental costs for children with diagnosed obesity using a top-down approach, until 2011, this area of research was strongly dominated by studies from the USA (12 of 21 studies). Most of these studies were based on data from different waves of the Medical Expenditure Panel Survey, and some were based on claims data. Whereas six US studies reported higher overall healthcare costs for obese children compared with normal-weight children, especially for children who were obese for 2 adjacent years, some studies reported increased expenditure only for subgroups, such as adolescents or girls, or only in single sectors of the healthcare system, such as prescription drugs or ambulatory or hospital costs. Only one of these earlier US studies did not find a significant association between obesity and higher healthcare costs. However, another study reported that total healthcare costs for the obese were not elevated before the age of 21 in females and before the age of 25 in males (for a review, see [3, 4]). In a recently published US study, Turer et al. analysed a 2005–2009 US medical expenditure panel survey sample of 10- to 17-year-old children and adolescents and found that obese children and adolescents had a greater risk of suboptimal health as well as greater use of prescriptions and emergency department visits. In contrast, obesity was not associated with more office visits or higher total expenditures [6]. It should be noted, however, that the analysis did not include the cost of inpatient health care services, which is often the cost-driving element in studies demonstrating increased expenditures for obese children .

After 2009, evidence on the economic burden of obesity in childhood has also been generated from other countries. A Canadian study reported no difference in physician costs between normal-weight and combined overweight/obese groups in 12 to 17 year-olds. In Israel, however, significantly higher medication expenditures as well as higher utilisation of paediatric clinics, hospitals and medication were found for obese children in a primary care centre. Two studies in Germany agree on significantly higher physician costs of obese children in different age groups. However, they differ in their findings concerning the costs for hospital and non-physician therapists. Only one study was found that additionally analysed indirect costs, i.e. productivity losses resulting from work absence of the parents due to illness of their child, which were higher for obese children (for a detailed review of these studies, see [3]). Aiming to complement this evidence base for Germany, another more recent study explored the association of BMI with the utilisation of pharmaceuticals and the related costs. The estimated drug costs were found to be 24% higher for obese children compared with the normal-weight group [7].

All of the above-mentioned studies analysed data from a study period of 1 to 2 years, and merely 3 studies examined the correlation between health care costs and weight status, using costs and/or BMI, over a longer time. A Canadian study observed that physician and hospital costs in the 3 years following their survey as well as physician costs from birth up to age 14 were significantly elevated for obese children compared with normal-weight children. Australian children who were overweight or obese at age 4–5 were shown to have higher pharmaceutical and non-hospital medical care costs during the following 5 years compared with normal-weight children. Additionally, the duration of overweight after age 5 was positively associated with later costs (for a detailed review, see [3]). The latest German study assessed the association between different patterns of BMI development from birth on and later healthcare utilisation and costs in children aged about 10. Costs were found to be doubled in the group with the most pronounced BMI growth (persistent rapid BMI-Standard Deviation Score growth up to age 5 years) compared to the group with a BMI development similar to the World Health Organization growth standards [8].

Discussion: Cost-of-Illness Studies

Our review has shown that almost all of the studies on the impact of childhood obesity on health care costs are bottom-up analyses. The evidence emerging from these studies is ambiguous. Some studies have found excess total health care costs for obesity, some only found excess costs for particular elements of health care, others only found excess costs for single subgroups of obese children, and some studies did not find any cost differences at all. Further empirical research should be devoted to efforts to identify the reasons producing the differences in the reported results. Possible explanations include differences in the statistical approaches applied to cost analyses, variation in the coverage of obesity-related services that are provided by different health care systems over time, age- and sex-dependent comorbid conditions and differences in the perception of health care needs based on social status.

Moreover, special consideration should be given to the question of to what extent do differences in the reference distributions of BMI as well as in the multiple cut-off points for the definition of overweight and obesity play a role in explaining the divergent findings. In addition, there is a still on-going discussion as to whether BMI should be used at all as an indicator of obesity, as BMI cannot differentiate between overweight due to increased muscle or fat mass. This holds true for studies on the economic burden of obesity, as there are studies demonstrating that e.g. waist circumference is a better predictor of current and future health care costs than BMI [9]. One study combined two approaches to define obesity, BMI and ICD codes, and found significantly higher costs for children with diagnosed obesity compared with the undiagnosed obese group (as defined by BMI) [10]. This finding might be an indication that severely obese children, who are not treated as a separate group in most analyses (mostly due to sample size reasons), are the main group of interest with respect to healthcare utilisation and thus are a particularly important target group for intervention.

Apart from the unknown reasons for the divergent study findings, there are two major limitations of the current research on the economic burden of childhood obesity. The first limitation results from the fact that the research is almost exclusively focused on the impact of obesity on health care expenditures, thus excluding all other components of direct and indirect costs. The most important among the neglected cost items is probably the cost accrued to unpaid caregivers of sick children, as time losses from work, household production or leisure activities because of the children's state of development and dependency can be considerable for parents and other informal caregivers.

The second limitation results from the short study period of most cost analyses, which rarely exceeded 2 years. It may be argued that a lifetime approach might be better suited to catch the long-term costs of obesity in children and adolescents. However, cohort studies of 10 or more years of follow-up are rare, and there is ample evidence from cost-of-illness studies in adults that obesity results in substantial excess cost over most of the life span. From a lifetime perspective, however, the negative impact of obesity on life expectancy may even lead to decreased total cost in obese persons [11].

Economic Evaluation of Interventions to Prevent or Manage Childhood Obesity

Cost-Effectiveness Studies: Methodological Aspects

Although a large body of evidence exists supporting effective interventions against childhood obesity, the mixed results from cost-of-illness studies leave some doubt as to whether all or most of them would be cost-saving within the time frame of a typical intervention study. High initial intervention costs may not be compensated by cost savings until much later; therefore, budget impact and short-term cost-effectiveness are relevant issues when judging new interventions. Cost-effectiveness is related to the concept of opportunity cost, which means that available health care resources should be spent in such a way that the optimal health outcomes are provided. Thus, comparing, for example, different prevention programmes, the more effective programme would be considered an acceptable alternative only if the difference in cost for a certain gain in effectiveness were below a threshold defined by societal consensus. An extensive methodological repertoire for cost-effectiveness analysis exists that includes different study types for short- and long-term horizons, methods to account for different types of uncertainty, and ways of valuing costs and outcomes that will occur at different times in the future.

Since randomised intervention trials usually have time horizons of at most a few years, any economic evaluation of childhood interventions over a relevant long-term horizon can only be done on the basis of decision models. Evidence from both approaches is needed, but it may not be directly comparable. In randomised trials, outcomes are often used that are directly related to obesity (e.g. anthropometric parameters), whereas long-term evaluations translate the intervention effects into health outcomes related to comorbidity and eventually into quality-adjusted life years (QALYs). In long-term evaluations, discounting is applied in order to account for the time preference of the decision makers. Thresholds for the society's willingness to pay for a certain intervention effect have been defined in some countries, but only with respect to life years or QALYs gained and not with respect to other outcome parameters.

Cost-Effectiveness of Prevention and Intervention Programmes: Results of Recent Studies

Evidence on the efficacy and effectiveness of obesity interventions in children and adolescents has been summarised in more than 30 reviews (e.g. [12, 13]). In contrast, few studies assessing their cost-effectiveness have been published.

One review included a total of 12 papers that were published in peer-reviewed journals until November 2009 and provided findings on the cost-effectiveness of interventions to prevent and manage obesity in childhood and adolescence [4]. Another review provided an update and identified 5 additional articles that were published until October 2011, including economic evaluations of 11 different programmes [3].

Of those 17 articles on a total of 23 different childhood obesity interventions, the majority was conducted as part of the Assessing Cost-Effectiveness in Obesity (ACE-Obesity) project in Australia (9 publications covering 15 programmes). This project applied a common economic evaluation methodology that was characterised by, among other things, a model-based cohort approach, a lifetime follow-up period, the use of 'current practice' as a comparator to the intervention under consideration and the use of disability-adjusted life years as a health outcome measure (for further details, see [14]). Of the remaining 8 studies, 5 were from the USA, and the rest were from New Zealand, Spain, and Finland.

The 17 publications included 12 school-based or joint school- and community-based preventive measures that were mainly targeted at all school children, independent of their weight status, in different age groups between 5 and 12 years. The school-based programmes followed various approaches: educational programmes aiming to improve nutrition and/or increase physical activity, physical activity programmes inside or outside the school, or programmes designed to achieve a change in school travel behaviour in favour of walking or cycling instead of going by car/bus. The 9 management interventions for already obese children included multi-disciplinary or general practice-based primary care programmes, family-based versus parent-only educational programmes, a pharmaceutical intervention targeted at obese children aged 12 to 16 years and a surgical intervention targeted at severely obese adolescents aged 14 to 19 years. Detailed information on the target population, selected methodological aspects and the cost-effectiveness results are presented elsewhere [3, 4].

Due to different methodologies regarding the economic evaluation, e.g. different health outcome measures, the comparability of the cost-effectiveness results is very limited. However, when looking at those studies which used comparable economic evaluation methods, the resulting incremental cost-effectiveness ratios (ICERs) vary considerably across the different interventions. There are, for example, two interventions – the Active After School Communities programme and the Travel SMART Schools programme – which are not cost-effective under base-case modelling assumptions when applying the usually accepted economic threshold levels [14]. At the other end of the range of ICERs, there are several ACE interventions with negative ICERs, indicating that under baseline assumptions, the cost-savings resulting from reducing the burden of disease attributable to obesity exceed the programme costs. When comparing population-based preventive interventions with targeted curative interventions, no clear picture emerges regarding their comparative efficiency. It should be noted, however, that the available evidence on the effectiveness of the interventions is of different quality, and therefore, a ranking of the programmes exclusively according to their estimated cost-effectiveness should be regarded with some caution (for a summary of the results, see [14]).

Since 2011, we have found two new studies in this area. One economic evaluation study analysed a structured, primary school-based programme in Germany that included health education, physical activity breaks and parental involvement. The results on cost-effectiveness were presented as EUR 11.11 per cm waist circumference prevented and EUR 18.55 per unit waist-to-height ratio prevented [15]. However, it is difficult to compare these results to other cost-effectiveness estimates due to the different outcome measures. Furthermore, when calculating cost-effectiveness, the authors of this study included only programme cost, and not potential short-term or long-term cost sequelae of reduced health risks due to decreased waist circumference or waist-to-height ratio. A recently published modelling study by Hollingworth et al. estimated the potential lifetime cost-effectiveness of 9 randomised controlled trial-evaluated lifestyle interventions (hospital- or community-based) to effectively treat overweight and obese children from the perspective of the UK National Health Service. For a hypothetical cohort of obese children aged 10–11 years, the discounted cost per life year gained was estimated as GBP 13,589 for an intervention that resulted in a median reduction in the BMI-Standard Deviation Score of 12 months at a moderate cost. The estimated results were similar for preventive interventions aimed at younger children and for interventions targeting obese and overweight children [16].

In addition to these evaluation studies, some model-based analyses trying to project short-term obesity outcomes into long-term health benefits of an intervention and to investigate which maximum amount of intervention cost would still meet acceptable standards of cost-effectiveness have been newly published [17–19]. One model was based on assumptions regarding lifetime healthcare costs and the persistence of obesity over time. Interventions yielding a 1% point reduction in obesity rate could achieve healthcare cost savings if the discounted intervention costs were between USD 280–339 per child for population-based interventions or between USD 1,648–2,735 for interventions that only targeted obese children. The results of the simulations indicated that targeted interventions could yield higher cost savings than population-based interventions for preschool children, whereas the opposite was the case for adolescents [18]. Wang et al. developed a BMI progression model and discovered that a 1% point reduction in both overweight and obesity rates in the study cohort would lower medical costs and considerably increase lifetime QALYs [17]. A similar study approach was applied by Trasande [19], who developed a mathematical model to predict the lifetime QALY gains and healthcare cost changes resulting from a 1% point reduction in the obesity rate in US children who were aged 12 in 2005. They concluded that an investment of USD 1,526 per overweight child could still produce an acceptable ICER [19].

However, the value of the information from these simulation studies should be regarded with caution. Due to differences in the data that were used and the assumptions that were made, these results are afflicted with large uncertainties, leading to considerable variations in the estimated results.

Discussion: Cost-Effectiveness of Interventions

To summarise, the currently available evidence from economic evaluations of childhood and adolescent obesity programmes support the expectation that preventive and management interventions with acceptable cost-effectiveness do exist. Some interventions even appear to be able to achieve health gains and save costs. It should be noted, however, that our limited knowledge about the persistence of BMI gains over time is an important source of uncertainty that needs to be reduced by appropriate follow-up studies.

Substantial differences in study design and measurement tools make it difficult to rank all evaluated interventions according to their comparative cost-effectiveness. Therefore, until now, it has been unclear whether preventive or treatment approaches are preferable in an economic perspective, and the most cost-effective time for preventive interventions during childhood and adolescence must be determined. It has even been speculated that postponing preventative action into early adulthood may be more cost-effective, due to the more immediate-occurring benefits of avoiding the otherwise high prevalence of obesity-related comorbidities that develop during adulthood [20].

Assessing the generalisability and transferability of the reported study results is also difficult, primarily due to a general lack of reporting contextual factors in intervention trials, which are critical for judging the relevance and applicability of findings in practice [21], as well as a lack of reporting programme fidelity and intervention integrity during implementation [22]. This assessment is urgently required to make more confident conclusions about the potential (cost-)effectiveness and successful dissemination of intervention evidence into different practice settings.

Altogether, the number of economic evaluation studies of childhood obesity prevention and intervention programmes is still relatively small compared to the large number of studies investigating their clinical effectiveness. Several study protocols have announced that further publications regarding the economic evaluation of childhood obesity prevention and treatment programmes may be expected soon, e.g. [23, 24]. New studies focusing on clinical effectiveness should facilitate future economic evaluations by at least collecting and reporting data on resource consumption caused by the implementation of the programmes under study. There are few examples for such a reporting of programme costs, two of which have been published recently. A Canadian study reported average costs per student of CAD 39 for a school-based programme managing to diminish the risk of overweight and obesity and to improve physical activity and dietary behaviour in class 5 students [25]. Another study estimated the costs for a community-based, non-health, professionally delivered programme (WATCH IT) within the English National Health Service that achieved significant reductions in overweight children at 6 months to be GBP 858 per child [26].

The results of economic evaluations of childhood obesity interventions are characterised by a large variation in ICERs, even among studies applying similar designs and measurements. This underscores the need for analysing the cost-effectiveness of those interventions in a standardised way to ensure the efficient allocation of resources that are available for improving children's health. However, economic evaluation of interventions to prevent or manage childhood obesity faces a number of challenges that should be addressed in future research in order to give the results more weight in decision-making (for a more detailed discussion, see [3]).

First, there are two contentious issues in the general health economic evaluation methodology that are of particular relevance to child obesity interventions. One is how to deal with health care costs in life-years gained, that are unrelated to obesity and its comorbidities. The current practice of excluding these costs may result in too-favourable efficiency estimates and feed an unfounded optimism among policy makers who tend to regard lifestyle interventions as cost-saving options. The other is the choice of the discount rate, which, due to the large time lag between the costs of the programme and its future health benefits and cost savings, can profoundly affect the results of economic evaluations. Therefore, the reasons for the choice of a specific number for this rate and its underlying rationale should be carefully made explicit in each evaluation [27].

Second, a decision-analytical modelling approach is required to evaluate child obesity interventions if the costs and health benefits are to be fully captured over the whole lifetime horizon. The hitherto used models appear to be rather simplistic, and some of their underlying assumptions may call their structural validity into question. For example, it is often assumed that an obesity intervention will produce health gains only via a decrease in BMI. However, there are other pathways by which those interventions may eventually lead to better health. A well-known example is the improvement of aerobic fitness due to increased physical activity, which predicts decreased morbidity and mortality independent of changes in BMI [28]. Considering those limitations of the currently available models, their further refinement appears to be feasible and desirable.

Third, there are various challenges regarding the economic evaluation of all child health interventions. Adopting a societal perspective requires inclusion of informal care activities in the costing exercise, which often play an important role in child health care. Until now, this has been rarely done, although appropriate valuation methods do exist. In addition, the strong inter-relationship in the quality of life among family members when a child is ill has led some investigators to argue that family members should be included in the economic evaluation, not only when measuring costs, but also when measuring benefits [29]. Furthermore, health state measurement and evaluation is hampered by a paucity of child-specific outcome measures with proven reliability and validity, particularly regarding preference-based measures, which, from an economist's point of view, are preferred because they support broad health care allocation decision-making across disease boundaries [29].

Fourth, most preventive obesity interventions are typical public health interventions, and evaluating those interventions raises specific methodological challenges [30]. First, these interventions include the proper identification, measurement and valuation of non-health targets, which, in the case of paediatric obesity interventions, may include aspects such as empowerment or strengthening the sense of community and self-confidence, which hints at the fact that evaluating the health impact and the cost-effectiveness of child obesity interventions usually cannot be more than single elements in a broader evaluation concept. Second, population-based interventions are often characterised by social diffusion effects into other non-targeted population groups. In a long-term research perspective, the suitability of transmission modelling approaches to catch those effects should be explored. Third, equity in health is often an issue of central concern in population-oriented public health interventions. Thus, in health economic evaluations, equity considerations should at least be considered in terms of narrative review.

Acknowledgements

This article was written as part of the Competence Network Obesity and was supported by the German Federal Ministry of Education and Research under grant number 01GI1127.

References

1 Ogden CL, Carroll MD, Kit BK, Flegal KM: Prevalence of childhood and adult obesity in the United States, 2011–2012. JAMA 2014;311:806–814.
2 Finkelstein EA, Ruhm CJ, Kosa KM: Economic causes and consequences of obesity. Annu Rev Public Health 2005;26:239–257.
3 John J, Wolfenstetter SB, Wenig CM: An economic perspective on childhood obesity: recent findings on cost of illness and cost effectiveness of interventions. Nutrition 2012;28:829–839.
4 John J, Wenig CM, Wolfenstetter SB: Recent economic findings on childhood obesity: cost-of-illness and cost-effectiveness of interventions. Curr Opin Clin Nutr Metab Care 2010;13:305–313.
5 Larg A, Moss JR: Cost-of-illness studies: a guide to critical evaluation. Pharmacoeconomics 2011;29:653–671.
6 Turer CB, Lin H, Flores G: Health status, emotional/behavioral problems, health care use, and expenditures in overweight/obese US children/adolescents. Acad Pediatr 2013;13:251–258.
7 Wenig CM, Knopf H, Menn P: Juvenile obesity and its association with utilisation and costs of pharmaceuticals–results from the KiGGS study. BMC Health Serv Res 2011;11:340.
8 Batscheider A, Rzehak P, Teuner CM, Wolfenstetter SB, Leidl R, von Berg A, Berdel D, Hoffmann B, Heinrich J, for the GINIplus and LISAplus Study Groups: Development of BMI values of German children and their healthcare costs. Econ Hum Biol 2014;12:56–66.
9 Hojgaard B, Gyrd-Hansen D, Olsen KR, Sogaard J, Sorensen TI: Waist circumference and body mass index as predictors of health care costs. PLoS One 2008;3:e2619.
10 Hampl SE, Carroll CA, Simon SD, Sharma V: Resource utilization and expenditures for overweight and obese children. Arch Pediatr Adolesc Med 2007;161:11–14.
11 van Baal PH, Polder JJ, de Wit GA, Hoogenveen RT, Feenstra TL, Boshuizen HC, Engelfriet PM, Brouwer WB: Lifetime medical costs of obesity: prevention no cure for increasing health expenditure. PLoS Med 2008;5:e29.
12 Safron M, Cislak A, Gaspar T, Luszczynska A: Effects of school-based interventions targeting obesity-related behaviors and body weight change: a systematic umbrella review. Behav Med 2011;37:15–25.
13 Hillier F, Pedley C, Summerbell C: Evidence base for primary prevention of obesity in children and adolescents. Bundesgesundheitsblatt Gesundheitsforschung Gesundheitsschutz 2011;54:259–264.
14 Victorian Government Department of Human Services: ACE-Obesity. Assessing cost-effectiveness of obesity interventions in children and adolescents: summary of results. 2006. http://www.health.vic.gov.au/healthpromotion/downloads/ace_obesity.pdf (accessed 2009).
15 Kesztyus D, Schreiber A, Wirt T, Wiedom M, Dreyhaupt J, Brandstetter S, Koch B, Wartha O, Muche R, Wabitsch M, Kilian R, Steinacker JM: Economic evaluation of URMEL-ICE, a school-based overweight prevention programme comprising metabolism, exercise and lifestyle intervention in children. Eur J Health Econ 2013;14:185–195.
16 Hollingworth W, Hawkins J, Lawlor DA, Brown M, Marsh T, Kipping RR: Economic evaluation of lifestyle interventions to treat overweight or obesity in children. Int J Obes (Lond) 2012;36:559–566.
17 Wang LY, Denniston M, Lee S, Galuska D, Lowry R: Long-term health and economic impact of preventing and reducing overweight and obesity in adolescence. J Adolesc Health 2010;46:467–473.
18 Ma S, Frick KD: A simulation of affordability and effectiveness of childhood obesity interventions. Acad Pediatr 2011;11:342–350.
19 Trasande L: How much should we invest in preventing childhood obesity? Health Aff (Millwood) 2010;29:372–378.

20 Cawley J: The cost-effectiveness of programs to prevent or reduce obesity: the state of the literature and a future research agenda. Arch Pediatr Adolesc Med 2007;161:611–614.
21 Klesges LM, Dzewaltowski DA, Glasgow RE: Review of external validity reporting in childhood obesity prevention research. Am J Prev Med 2008;34:216–223.
22 Walter U, Pott E, Kliche T: On the importance of reporting public health programmes. J Public Health 2011;19:281–282.
23 Hesketh KD, Campbell K, Salmon J, McNaughton SA, McCallum Z, Cameron A, Ball K, Gold L, Andrianopoulos N, Crawford D: The Melbourne Infant Feeding, Activity and Nutrition Trial (InFANT) Program follow-up. Contemp Clin Trials 2013;34:145–151.
24 Robertson W, Stewart-Brown S, Stallard N, Petrou S, Griffiths F, Thorogood M, Simkiss D, Lang R, Reddington K, Poole F, Rye G, Khan KA, Hamborg T, Kirby J: Evaluation of the effectiveness and cost-effectiveness of Families for Health V2 for the treatment of childhood obesity: study protocol for a randomized controlled trial. Trials 2013;14:81.
25 Ohinmaa A, Langille JL, Jamieson S, Whitby C, Veugelers PJ: Costs of implementing and maintaining comprehensive school health: the case of the Annapolis Valley Health Promoting Schools program. Can J Public Health 2011;102:451–454.
26 Spoor C, Sahota P, Wellings C, Rudolf MC: Costing a pilot complex community-based childhood obesity intervention. J Hum Nutr Diet 2013;26:126–131.
27 Schad M, John J: Towards a social discount rate for the economic evaluation of health technologies in Germany: an exploratory analysis. Eur J Health Econ 2012;13:127–144.
28 Blair SN, Kohl HW 3rd, Barlow CE, Paffenbarger RS Jr, Gibbons LW, Macera CA: Changes in physical fitness and all-cause mortality. A prospective study of healthy and unhealthy men. JAMA 1995;273:1093–1098.
29 Ungar WJ: Challenges in health state valuation in paediatric economic evaluation: are QALYs contraindicated? Pharmacoeconomics 2011;29:641–652.
30 Weatherly H, Drummond M, Claxton K, Cookson R, Ferguson B, Godfrey C, Rice N, Sculpher M, Sowden A: Methods for assessing the cost-effectiveness of public health interventions: key challenges and recommendations. Health Policy 2009;93:85–92.

Prof. Dr. Rolf Holle
Helmholtz Zentrum München, German Research Center for Environmental Health
Institute of Health Economics and Health Care Management
Ingolstädter Landstrasse 1
DE–85764 Neuherberg (Germany)
E-Mail holle@helmholtz-muenchen.de

Kiess W, Wabitsch M, Maffeis C, Sharma AM (eds): Metabolic Syndrome and Obesity in Childhood and Adolescence.
Pediatr Adolesc Med. Basel, Karger, 2015, vol 19, pp 160–165 (DOI: 10.1159/000368127)

Prevention of Childhood and Adolescent Obesity and its Barriers

Jana Markert

IFB AdiposityDiseases, Medical Faculty, University of Leipzig, Leipzig, Germany

Abstract

The high prevalence of childhood and adolescent obesity and the existence of an obesogenic environment in industrialized countries demand a societal obesity prevention strategy, i.e. structured health promotion. As scientists demand 'far bigger and bolder steps' in the field of pediatric obesity prevention, this issue has to move into public focus. The present societal infrastructures in industrialized countries are apparently obesogenic, i.e. a societal environment that generates overweight and obesity-promoting behavior. In an obesogenic environment, leading a healthy lifestyle becomes an every day life challenge that expends personal resources (e.g. knowledge, time, finances, self-efficacy). Nevertheless, several possibilities exist to make an industrialized consumer society less obesogenic. Putting this approach into practice requires a public will in order to convince political decision makers and involved stakeholders on all societal levels. Therefore, the main scientific task for the future should not only be to produce verifiable research outcomes but to communicate the obtained results outside of the scientific community in order to develop a societal rethinking about health prevention.

Prevention of Childhood and Adolescent Obesity

The epidemic dimension of obesity and its comorbidities (e.g. metabolic syndrome) requires the prevention of further incidences. Public health science defines three different levels of prevention: universal prevention and health promotion, selective prevention, and targeted prevention. In this chapter, these three terms and their connection to pediatric obesity will be illustrated.

Universal Prevention and Health Promotion

This level of prevention is directed to the whole population, independent of a person's weight status, in order to counteract an increase in obesity prevalence within that population. The most common method used here is the spreading of cognitive information. Universal prevention is usually provided by federal or federally funded institutions in the form of TV advertising, information leaflets, websites, and merchandizing material like buttons, stickers, and posters.

Selective Prevention

Selective prevention aims to address the persons at risk. The scientific literature describes several risk factors for pediatric obesity, e.g. low socio-economic status, obese parents (especially obese mothers), single parenthood, abnormal birth weight, genetic predisposition, etc. Selective prevention measures only address these vulnerable groups.

Targeted Prevention

Targeted obesity prevention directs its efforts toward already affected persons within the field of pediatric obesity rather than toward families and single-parent children or adolescents in order to hinder a further increase in body weight.

Behavioral and Environmental Prevention

In addition to the described prevention levels, the following two modes of prevention, which are applicable to all three prevention levels, have to be considered: behavioral and environmental prevention.

Behavioral prevention acts on the micro level. It addresses the individual person or the individual family and demands a change in health behavior. In contrast, environmental prevention acts on the macro level of prevention by creating health-promoting living spaces/surroundings that are accessible to the whole population instead of only to targeted persons or families. Interventions targeting the combination of environments and upstream determinants as well as those involving the whole community appear to be more effective than those that focus on education by simply targeting only children or families [1].

Barriers within the Prevention of Childhood and Adolescent Obesity

Barriers of the Target Group

The scientific literature presents many factors that hinder parents from taking action to change their family lifestyle into a healthier one. Authors describe time constraints in families with overweight children [2], and as most affected families posses a low socio-economic status (SES) [3], financial constraints are also obvious. In addition, a lack of parental awareness of their child's weight status is described [4].

Another publication revealed that families with pediatric obesity have great expectations toward other involved persons and institutions. They attribute a mediating role to the involved physician, and they expect schools to educate their kids in healthy behavior. Overall, these parents do not show confidence in their own abilities to manage the weight status of their child [5].

Barriers for Academic Research

In a review on childhood obesity prevention, the authors stated that 'effective action requires an evidence base' [6], and this statement is absolutely true. Academic research has already built up an evidence base for obesity prevention by proving the effectiveness of different single parameters that are required to create a less obesogenic environment. One can find 'classic' factors such as a negative correlation between weight status and high media time [7], and the same correlation was shown toward low physical activity [8], sweetened beverages [9–11], and high dietary fat [12]. Also, the influence of the neighborhood environment on the weight status of an individual has been evaluated, and a negative correlation between the socio-economic status of a living area and the habitants' weight status was shown in a complex housing experiment [13].

Now, the effectiveness of the combined parameters needs to be evaluated. So far, the obesity prevention programs that have taken place have been limited in time and setting (e.g. 1- or 2-year prevention programs in elementary schools), apparently due to funding, feasibility, and last but not least data analysis. Foremost, funding is often restricted in time (normally up to 2 or 3 years and rarely longer) and amount. Ensuring the yearlong realization of such a complex program, accompanied by the participation of several scientists from different disciplines in the performance and data evaluation, requires a lot of financial investment. As the distribution of financial resources toward an issue depends on the importance associated with that issue by funding bodies, more political work has to be done by researchers within the field of health promotion. Next, feasibility also shows diverse facets. First, it is not feasible to involve all potential stakeholders in an area all at once. Second, the time needed to really show preventive effects has to be counted in decades. Third, it is critical to find a matching community-level comparison group in which no health-promoting effects have been allowed for decades. In addition, scientific data analysis is ambitious, as a mixture of different methods and scales for measuring changes in the potential obesogenic parameters and in the outcome variable (prevalence of overweight and obesity) has to be determined at the start of the program.

In the short term, assessing the effectiveness of obesity prevention is problematic due to its complex nature [1]. Therefore, it is recommended for researchers to work closely with practitioners and policy makers as well as outside the scope of traditional funding infrastructures [14]. At times, it has seemed as if academic research has stood still at the point that Hill stated in 1998 that 'a [...] barrier is the *perception* that we not know how to prevent obesity' [15].

Barriers within a Consumer Society

Industrialized consumer societies show high prevalence rates of overweight and obesity. These communities are shaped by different stakeholders (government, health insurances, industries, media, general public), which sometime pursue different goals with regard to pediatric obesity.

The government of a country has a fiduciary duty to the health and welfare of the population of that country. Health insurances show a commercial interest in the health of citizens. Industries (e.g. food industries, electronic industries, pharmaceutical industries) want to sell their products to all potential consumer groups and are supported by commercial advertising. The media aim to share their (sometimes divergent) information and are funded by the commercial advertising of the industries. The general public freely makes its decisions according to its priorities, its intellect, and its personal resources.

Within this context of competing interests regarding the market of health promotion, it is not surprising that the subjective assessment of a family's health behavior often totally differs from the suggestions of experts and health professionals [16]. So, in fact, it is difficult for target families to develop a subjective need for action [17], and without the latter, an improvement in health behavior is impossible.

The Potential for a Shift from Behavioral to Environmental Prevention

The present societal infrastructures in industrialized countries are apparently obesogenic, i.e. a societal environment has developed that generates overweight- and obesity-promoting behavior. Individuals with the corresponding genetic disposition and metabolic characteristics have an increased probability of becoming obese compared to persons without this inherited predisposition. In an obesogenic environment, leading a healthy lifestyle becomes an every day life challenge that expends personal resources (e.g. knowledge, time, finances, self-efficacy). These resources often are limited for vulnerable families at risk for childhood obesity (low educational background, single-parenthood, low household-net-income, low self-efficacy-acceptance, etc.), making the long-term implementation of a healthy lifestyle difficult or even impossible.

If universal prevention and health promotion turned away from the exclusive transfer of responsibility onto the obese individual toward the development of area-wide health-promoting infrastructures, the sustainable implementation of a healthy lifestyle could be an easy choice for every individual, independent of their genetic and metabolic configuration and weight status.

Shifting the focus of responsibility for childhood obesity away from target individuals toward the environment in order to solve the societal problem of childhood obesity has been suggested by researchers all over the world for over 15 years [15, 18–21]. However, until now, no method for the long-term implementation of societal lifestyle changes has been determined.

The most difficult part seems to be to bringing together the different pressure groups of this problem, i.e. public authorities, health professionals, industries, health insurances, educational establishment, and media, in order to make a long-term orientation toward health promotion possible. Doing so will only work with a public will and with public pressure, as not all involved stakeholders feel an intrinsic attitude toward universal obesity prevention and health promotion.

Conclusion

Every person must have the chance to sustainably implement a healthy lifestyle into their everyday life, regardless of the social context. Therefore, societal changes in universal obesity prevention and health promotion are needed and could bring together the parameters of obesity prevention measures that are proven to be effective. The realization of this approach requires a public will in order to convince political decision makers and involved stakeholders on all societal levels. The main scientific task for the future should not only be to produce verifiable research outcomes but also to communicate the obtained results outside of the scientific community to enable the development of a societal rethinking about health prevention.

References

1 Hillier F, Pedley C, Summerbell C: Evidence base for primary prevention of obesity in children and adolescents. Bundesgesundheitsbl 2011;54:259–264.

2 Alff F, Markert J, Zschaler S, Gausche R, Kiess W, Blüher S: Reasons for (non)participation in a telephone-based intervention programme for families with overweight children. PLoS ONE 2012;7:e34580.

3 Danielzik S, Czerwinski-Mast M, Langnaese K, Dilba B, Müller MJ: Parental overweight, socioeconomic status and high birth weight are the major determinants of overweight and obesity in 5- to 7-year-old children: baseline data of the Kiel Obesity Prevention Study (KOPS). Int J Obes 2004;28:1494–1502.

4 Markert J, Alff F, Zschaler S, Gausche R, Kiess W, Blüher S: Prevention of childhood obesity: recruiting strategies via local paediatricians and study protocol for a telephone-based counselling programme. Obes Res Clin Pract 2013;7:e476–e486.

5 Booth ML, King LA, Pagnini DL, Wilkenfeld RL, Booth SL: Parents of school students on childhood overweight: the Weight of Opinion Study. J Paediatr Child Health 2009;45:194–198.

6 Birch LL, Ventura AK: Preventing childhood obesity: what works? Int J Obes 2009;33:S74-S81.

7 Toschke AM, Rückinger S, Böhler E, Von Kries R: Adjusted population attributable fractions and preventable potential risk factors for childhood obesity. Public Health Nutr 2007;10:902–906.

8 Parsons TJ, Power C, Manor O: Physical activity, television viewing and body mass index: a cross-sectional analysis from childhood to adulthood in the 1958 British cohort. Int J Obes Relat Metab Disord 2005;29:1212–1221.

9 Fung C, McIsaac J-LD, Kuhle S, Kirk SFL, Veugelers PJ: The impact of a population-level school food and nutrition policy on dietary intake and body weights of Canadian children. Prev Med 2013;57:934–940.

10 Muckelbauer R, Libuda L, Clausen K, Toschke AM, Reinehr T, Kersting M: Promotion and provision of drinking water in schools for overweight prevention: randomized, controlled cluster trial. Pediatrics 2009; 123:e661–e667.

11 James J, Thomas P, Cavan D, Kerr D: Preventing childhood obesity by reducing consumption of carbonated drinks: cluster randomised controlled trial. BMJ 2004;328:1236–1241.

12 Foreyt JP, Poston WS: Consensus view on the role of dietary fat and obesity. Am J Med 2002;113:60–62.

13 Ludwig J, Sanbonmatsu L, Gennetian L, Adam E, Duncan GJ, Katz LF, Kessler RC, Kling JR, Lindau ST, Whitaker RC, McDade TW: Neighborhoods, obesity, and diabetes – a randomized social experiment. N Engl J Med 2011;365:1509–1519.

14 Raine KD, Plotnikoff R, Nykiforuk C, Deegan H, Hemphill E, Storey K, Schopflocher D, Veugelers P, Wild TC, Ohinmaa A: Reflections on community-based population health intervention and evaluation for obestity and chronic disease prevention: the Healthy Alberta Communities project. Int J Public Health 2010;55:679–686.
15 Hill JO, Peters JC: Environmental contributions to the obesity epidemic. Science 1998;280:1371–1374.
16 Adamo KB, Papadakis S, Dojeiji L, Turnau M, Simmons L, Parameswaran M, Cunningham J, Pipe AL, Reid RD: Using path analysis to understand parents' perceptions of their children's weight, physical activity and eating habits in the Champlain region of Ontario. Paediatr Child Health 2010;15:e33–e41.
17 Finne E, Reinehr T, Schaefer A, Winkel K, Kolip P: Overweight children and adolescents – is there a subjective need for treatment? Int J Public Health 2009;54:112–116.
18 Schwartz MB, Puhl R: Childhood obesity: a societal problem to solve. Obes Rev 2003;4:57–71.
19 Summerbell CD, Waters E, Edmunds L, Kelly S, Brown T, Campbell KJ: Interventions for preventing obesity in children. Cochrane Database Syst Rev 2005;(3):CD001871.
20 Swinburn BA, Sacks G, Hall KD, McPherson K, Finegood DT, Moodie ML, Gortmaker SL: The global obesity pandemic: shaped by global drivers and local environments. Lancet 2011;378:804–814.
21 Gortmaker SL, Swinburn BA, Levy D, Carter R, Mabry PL, Finegood DT, Huang T, Marsh T, Moodie ML: Changing the future of obesity: science, policy, and action. Lancet 2011;378:838–847.

Jana Markert
IFB AdiposityDiseases, Medical Faculty, University of Leipzig
Philipp-Rosenthal-Strasse 27, Haus M
DE–04103 Leipzig (Germany)
E-Mail Jana.Markert@medizin.uni-leipzig.de

Kiess W, Wabitsch M, Maffeis C, Sharma AM (eds): Metabolic Syndrome and Obesity in Childhood and Adolescence.
Pediatr Adolesc Med. Basel, Karger, 2015, vol 19, pp 166–170 (DOI: 10.1159/000368133)

E-Health in Overweight and Obesity Prevention

Sabine Herget

IFB AdiposityDiseases, Medical Faculty, University of Leipzig, Leipzig, Germany

Abstract

Obesity prevention based on electronic technology has attracted increased attention over the last few years. Due to their relatively high computer literacy, children and adolescents are the main target group for these health promotion programs delivered through new media. Programs should be directed at various levels (micro, meso, and community) to target pediatric obesity and metabolic syndrome. Furthermore, they need to be based on health psychological frameworks and have to incorporate interactive components. The participation rates of programs need to be carefully monitored. Factors hindering or facilitating program implementation need to be continuously examined for the optimization of future research programs. Family and school-based settings for the delivery of internet-based prevention programs seem to be most effective. However, community approaches also need further attention via research and translation into practice.

Prevention, E-Learning, and the Internet

Prevention of metabolic syndrome and obesity in childhood and adolescence is a crucial goal, as obesity and associated diseases continue into adulthood and lead to considerable public health and economic costs [1, 2]. As described in the previous section, prevention of pediatric obesity and metabolic syndrome implicates certain barriers, which are handled by applying new preventive efforts, including the application of new media, in addition to other approaches.

Due to their acquisition of computer literacy early in life, children and adolescents are a major target group of new media campaigns. Public health organizations have also begun using this channel as a new form of low-threshold delivery of health-promoting messages and information [3, 4].

To simplify the complex structure of e-health campaigns targeting prevention of obesity and metabolic syndrome, this chapter describes different settings in which e-health based programs are applied as preventive measures. The programs can either address children and adolescents directly or parents and immediate caregivers as well as the meso-level environment, including educational settings and health care.

E-Health Prevention at the Micro Level

Health-promoting strategies targeted at children and adolescents in their home setting are on the rise. However, very few programs are directed at very young children alone, as their immediate environments, including parents, provide necessary enablers of healthy behavior and are often regarded as 'agents of change' [5]. Previous interventions directly addressing children implemented websites or CD-ROM games offering weekly modules containing *role modelling, problem solving, and goal setting* to promote fruit and vegetable intake and increases in physical activity [6]. When applying e-health-based programs addressed to children in their home environment, it is absolutely necessary to monitor log-on and program attrition rates and to find a theoretical basis for the design of the intervention in order to improve evidence-based e-health learning for obesity prevention.

Adolescents are often directly addressed by programs focusing on prevention of obesity or metabolic syndrome. The program contents include the promotion of physical activity to increase fruit and vegetable consumption as well as psychosocial management. The technologies applied range from internet websites to CD-ROM games, text messages, and mobile phone applications ('apps'). Interventions solely focusing on *internet websites* for adolescents may comprise methods such as *psycho-educational lessons, discussion groups, tailored feedback,* or *lessons with a gaming approach* [6]. In particular, interactive components were found to be appealing, as they motivated participants to learn by example and experience. The involvement of social media is a controversial subject. However, social networks could facilitate broad implementation of interventions [7, 8].

Mobile phone apps are also becoming increasingly popular for health promotion among adolescents, as most youngsters own a smartphone and especially because at-risk or underserved groups possess access to new mobile phone technology [9]. Expert-recommended strategies, available via apps on the market for adolescents, are *BMI follow-ups over time, assessment of motivation to change in behavior, tailored strategies for goal setting, examination of environmental influences, involvement of the family setting,* and *a combination of multiple behavior changes* [10]. However, evidence-based practices need to be incorporated into commercially available apps for adolescent users to actually increase the likelihood of effective health promotion.

In addition to smartphone applications, even the use of text messages and phone calls is an effective and very personal way to deliver health promotion messages to adolescents. Interventions can also be complemented by text message reminders to lower attrition rates [11].

To date, other social media, such as social networks, have rarely been used as the sole component of health promotion programs but are commonly used to raise awareness of health promotion programs. Overall, prevention programs focusing directly on children and adolescents should be based on a theoretical framework for behavior change and incorporate interactive media components to engage the target group in active learning and to build motivation to make sustainable lifestyle changes.

E-Health Prevention at the Meso Level: Parents and the Family Setting
Recent studies revealed that the internet and the phone are good channels through which to address the whole family, and especially parents, for obesity prevention in childhood and adolescence [12]. Parental and family involvement helps to enforce health behavior change and increases the sustainability of programs for designing a healthy home environment for children [13]. Health information is also a topic often researched on the internet by adults. Even low health literacy among parents can be overcome by designing an appealing *website with multiple layers of content and incorporating audio and video sources* [14].

Research has shown that family-based interventions enabling healthy lifestyle behaviors are effective when using evidence-based approaches such as *goal setting, self-monitoring,* and *involvement of parents' health behavior.* The contents of internet interventions delivered to parents can comprise *advice, self-assessment, feedback, awareness raising, and motivation regarding parenting style and self-efficacy* [6, 12].

Tailoring e-health and phone interventions according to parents' and the family's needs and habits can further increase program adherence by respecting individually relevant topics related to health behavior change [15, 16].

E-Health Prevention at the Meso Level: Education and the Health Care System

School-based internet obesity prevention programs have led to improvement of the health behavior of children in the short term. Generally, the school setting can be recommended for the implementation of internet prevention measures because the level of outreach, even to elevated-risk groups, is high and because distribution can be widespread. Most internet programs comprise *educational lessons, goal setting, skill building, incentives, tailored feedback, stage-of-change-based or tailored advice, and assessment of health behavior* to change nutrition or physical activity habits. Implementation and effective outreach are often dependent not only on motivational factors but also on teachers' acceptance of the program and the school environment in general. It has also been found that print-based programs remain almost equally as effective as internet-based programs [17].

Generally, there is a high number of school-based e-health programs focusing on obesity prevention and health promotion, but actual effects have only been documented for short follow-up periods. Participation rates decline over time, and implementation is often dependent on the school curriculum and teachers' perception and involvement. To translate science into practice, future studies need to examine process implementation, participation, and attrition rates in relation to the outcomes of preventive interventions.

In addition to school-based interventions, health care settings can also serve as indirect implementation targets for prevention of metabolic syndrome. Currently, educational lessons delivered to general practitioners, nurses, and other health care workers are often delivered through e-learning modules and thereby help to increase awareness, knowledge, and skills to prevent the onset of obesity in childhood and adolescence [18, 19].

Conclusions

Electronic technology can be used for the large-scale and low-cost delivery of health promotion programs for both children/adolescents and their environment. The availability of technology is widespread, and therefore, outreach, even to at-risk populations, is absolutely possible. However, programs need to monitor participation rates and act against attrition. The incorporation of interactive lessons, face-to-face counselling, or the involvement of a community setting would be favorable to increase the effectiveness and sustainability of prevention programs based on new media technologies.

References

1 Herouvi D, Karanasios E, Karayianni C, Karavanaki K: Cardiovascular disease in childhood: the role of obesity. Eur J Pediatr 2013;172:721–732.

2 Halfon N, Verhoef PA, Kuo AA: Childhood antecedents to adult cardiovascular disease. Pediatr Rev 2012;33:51–60; quiz 61.

3 Hillier F, Pedley C, Summerbell C: Evidence base for primary prevention of obesity in children and adolescents. Bundesgesundheitsblatt Gesundheitsforschung Gesundheitsschutz 2011;54:259–264.

4 Bundeszentrale für gesundheitliche Aufklärung: Kinderübergewicht. 2014. http://www.bzga-kinderuebergewicht.de/ (accessed February 5, 2014).

5 Faith MS, Van Horn L, Appel LJ, Burke LE, Carson JA, et al: Evaluating parents and adult caregivers as 'agents of change' for treating obese children: evidence for parent behavior change strategies and research gaps: a scientific statement from the American Heart Association. Circulation 2012; 125:1186–1207.

6 Nguyen B, Kornman KP, Baur LA: A review of electronic interventions for prevention and treatment of overweight and obesity in young people. Obes Rev 2011;12:e298–e314.

7 Li JS, Barnett TA, Goodman E, Wasserman RC, Kemper AR: Approaches to the prevention and management of childhood obesity: the role of social networks and the use of social media and related electronic technologies: a scientific statement from the American Heart Association. Circulation 2013; 127:260–267.

8 Maher CA, Lewis LK, Ferrar K, Marshall S, De Bourdeaudhuij I, et al: Are health behavior change interventions that use online social networks effective? A systematic review. J Med Internet Res 2014;16:e40.

9 Thomas S, Heinrich S, Kuhnlein A, Radon K: The association between socioeconomic status and exposure to mobile telecommunication networks in children and adolescents. Bioelectromagnetics 2010;31: 20–27.

10 Schoffman DE, Turner-McGrievy G, Jones SJ, Wilcox S: Mobile apps for pediatric obesity prevention and treatment, healthy eating, and physical activity promotion: just fun and games? Transl Behav Med 2013;3:320–325.

11 Hebden L, Balestracci K, McGeechan K, Denney-Wilson E, Harris M, et al: 'TXT2BFiT' a mobile phone-based healthy lifestyle program for preventing unhealthy weight gain in young adults: study protocol for a randomized controlled trial. Trials 2013;14:75.
12 Hohman KH, Price SN, Sonneville K, Rifas-Shiman SL, Gortmaker SL, et al: Can the internet be used to reach parents for family-based childhood obesity interventions? Clin Pediatr (Phila) 2012;51:314–320.
13 Verloigne M, Van Lippevelde W, Maes L, Brug J, De Bourdeaudhuij I: Family- and school-based correlates of energy balance-related behaviours in 10- to 12-year-old children: a systematic review within the ENERGY (EuropeaN Energy balance Research to prevent excessive weight Gain among Youth) project. Public Health Nutr 2012;15:1380–1395.
14 Mackert M, Kahlor L, Tyler D, Gustafson J: Designing e-health interventions for low-health-literate culturally diverse parents: addressing the obesity epidemic. Telemed J E Health 2009;15:672–677.
15 Markert J, Alff F, Zschaler S, Gausche R, Kiess W, et al: Prevention of childhood obesity: recruiting strategies via local paediatricians and study protocol for a telephone-based counselling programme. Obes Res Clin Pract 2013;7:e476–e486.
16 Morrison LG, Yardley L, Powell J, Michie S: What design features are used in effective e-health interventions? A review using techniques from Critical Interpretive Synthesis. Telemed J E Health 2012;18: 137–144.
17 Whittemore R, Chao A, Popick R, Grey M: School-based internet obesity prevention programs for adolescents: a systematic literature review. Yale J Biol Med 2013;86:49–62.
18 Ruggeri K, Farrington C, Brayne C: A global model for effective use and evaluation of e-learning in health. Telemed J E Health 2013;19:312–321.
19 Rudolf MC, Hunt C, George J, Hajibagheri K, Blair M: HENRY: development, pilot and long-term evaluation of a programme to help practitioners work more effectively with parents of babies and pre-school children to prevent childhood obesity. Child Care Health Dev 2010;36:850–857.

Sabine Herget
IFB AdiposityDiseases, Medical Faculty, University of Leipzig
Philipp-Rosenthal-Strasse 27, Haus M
DE–04103 Leipzig (Germany)
E-Mail Sabine.Herget@medizin.uni-leipzig.de

Kiess W, Wabitsch M, Maffeis C, Sharma AM (eds): Metabolic Syndrome and Obesity in Childhood and Adolescence.
Pediatr Adolesc Med. Basel, Karger, 2015, vol 19, pp 171–178 (DOI: 10.1159/000368134)

Obesity Treatment Programmes

Thomas Reinehr

Department of Paediatric Endocrinology, Diabetes and Nutrition Medicine, Vestische Hospital for Children and Adolescents, University of Witten/Herdecke, Datteln, Germany

Abstract

The efficiency of obesity treatment programmes based on diet, exercise and behaviour therapy in obese children and adolescents, especially when parents are involved, has been proven by several randomised controlled trials and meta-analyses. A stable weight in growing children is known to be associated with an improvement in cardiovascular risk factors and comorbidities of obesity. In clinical practice, the degree of weight loss due to obesity treatment programmes is only moderate, and these interventions are successful only in a subgroup of obese children. In particular, young children and less-overweight children profit from obesity treatment programmes. Failures in weight reduction are not only attributed to lack of motivation and willingness to change behaviour but also to genetic background and adaptive hormonal changes, which result in a reduced resting metabolic rate and increased hunger. Therefore, blaming obese children and their parents for unsuccessful weight loss is inadequate. There is still a great need for high-quality, multi-centre trials with long-term follow-up that are aimed to enhance obesity treatment programmes by improving the techniques used and the education of therapists.

Introduction

Obesity treatment programmes based on lifestyle intervention are recommended as the primary treatment for childhood obesity [1–3]. These interventions are usually comprised of diet and exercise interventions using behavioural therapy techniques [3, 4]. In the following sections, the knowledge concerning these treatment modalities are presented, and the limitations of obesity treatment programmes are highlighted.

Diet

While years ago, weight reduction in children was based on strict dietary concepts (for example, energy intake limited to 1,000 or 1,500 calories per day), this approach has been discontinued for several reasons: strict caloric guidelines cannot be adhered to for longer periods of time and the families do not learn to change their daily routine dietary intake [5]. Furthermore, a hypocaloric diet in children jeopardises growth and development by deficiencies in essential vitamins and minerals. In addition, energy consumption differs widely, even between children of the same age and gender [6]. The genetic background and individual physical activity as well as other factors determine caloric need; therefore, most lifestyle interventions try to reduce individual calorie intake by about 30%, even if studies proving this approach are lacking [3, 4].

Currently, there is debate as to whether a low-fat (usually 30% of calories as fat) or a low-carbohydrate diet is more efficacious [1]. At the present time, there is insufficient paediatric evidence to warrant recommending any one diet over another. The only effective diet advice proven by randomised controlled trials (RCTs) is a reduction of sweetened drink intake [7, 8]. Furthermore, a reduction of fast food intake also seems promising because consumption of fast food is a well-known predictor of weight gain, as demonstrated in prospective studies [2].

Exercise Treatment

Sport sessions to improve physical activity are a widely used component of obesity treatment programmes for children and adolescents. The aims of these sessions are to improve self-confidence and acquire a positive body image, to improve aerobic and anaerobic fitness as well as muscle strength, and therefore to reduce body weight without the loss of lean body mass. Sports activities are well accepted by obese children if they are performed in closed groups that exclude normal-weight children [2].

However, meta-analyses and many RCTs of physical activity interventions found no effect of these sessions on the BMI of obese children [3, 4]. Additionally, increasing daily physical activity by walking to school or kindergarten instead of using cars or buses was not associated with a significant weight loss in RCT studies [2]. On the other hand, increased physical activity was associated with an improvement of fitness and cardiovascular risk factors in obese children, even without weight loss [2].

In recent years, many interventions have focused on sedentary behaviour by reducing media time to treat childhood obesity. The results of the meta-analysis and RCTs focused on reducing sedentary activity demonstrated both favourable and unfavourable impacts on weight status [2, 4]. The most promising results were seen in preschool children [9].

Behaviour Therapy

Successful obesity treatment programmes are frequently based on behaviour therapy, including impulse control techniques, self-instruction, cognitive restructuring, development of problem-solving strategies, behaviour contracts, booster systems, self-reflection curves, and model learning via parents [2]. The effectiveness of behaviour therapy approaches has been proven in several RCT studies and meta-analyses [10]. In recent years, interventions for obese children have moved to systemic and solution-focused theories as well as family therapy [11] and include avoiding blaming and highlighting strengths instead of weaknesses. Motivational interviewing has been advocated as an especially useful technique to increase motivation [12].

Setting and Duration of Obesity Treatment Programmes

Successful interventions lasted 6–12 months, but no RCT demonstrated that a short-term intervention over 2–8 weeks achieved long-term success at a 12-month follow-up [3, 4]. Most weight reduction programmes are provided by outpatient clinics [3, 4], and obesity intervention programmes in schools failed to achieve weight loss [2]. A new medium for intervention is the Internet. However, interventions via Internet for obese adolescents have failed to reduce BMI [2]. In addition, telephone coaching and electronic contact interventions were not associated with changes of BMI in obese children [2].

Successful obesity treatment programmes were always performed as group treatment [3, 4], which could be more cost-effective than individual approaches. Furthermore, motivation could be increased through interactions with the group participants.

Target Group of Obesity Intervention Programmes

While obesity treatment programmes 10 years ago focused on children and adolescents, it has become quite clear in recent years that interventions involving parents are more effective than interventions solely involving obese children or adolescents [1–4]. This fact likely explains the limited effect of inpatient, school, Internet, and telephone settings. Parents control the health behaviour of their children and have an important model function for the eating and exercise behaviour of their children.

Side Effects of Obesity Treatment Programmes

While growth failure during weight loss due to obesity intervention programmes has been excluded, some studies have reported eating disorders associated with lifestyle intervention (for details, see [3]). If children drop out of lifestyle intervention or fail to lose weight, their self-confidence may be reduced because the obese child 'learns' that she/he cannot change his/her weight.

Effectiveness of Obesity Treatment Programmes

Meta-analyses summarising the findings of >60 RCTs with >5,500 children reported that obesity treatment programmes are effective in reducing obesity, in contrast to standard care or self-help [3, 4]. Interestingly, quality of life improves in obese children participating in obesity treatment programmes independent of the degree of weight loss [2].

In general, the degree of weight reduction and the success rate of obesity treatment programmes are higher in children compared to adults [2–4, 13]. The mean reduction of standard deviation score of BMI (BMI-SDS) of obesity treatment programmes for obese children 12 months after onset of intervention ranged from –0.2 to –0.6 BMI-SDS, with better results for children aged 8–12 who were less overweight [2–4].

Interestingly, one study in the literature has analysed the impact of lifestyle intervention on overweight but not obese children [14]. The success rate in this study was very high (92%), even 1 year after the end of the 6-month intervention period [14]. However, further independent and larger studies are needed to prove this promising outcome. On the other hand, obesity treatment programmes were not successful in extremely obese adolescents [2].

Only very few studies in children analysed the changes in weight status ≥5 years after the end of treatment [2, 4]. All of these studies reported that the achieved weight loss due to intervention was sustained for 5–10 years, in contrast to studies in adults that reported weight regain in the majority of the participants [13].

From a medical point of view, improvement of cardiovascular risk factors and comorbidities of obesity are the primary aims of obesity treatment programmes. Already, a decrease of BMI-SDS ≥0.25 has been associated with improvements in cardiovascular risk factors, intima-media thickness, androgen excess in polycystic ovary syndrome and non-alcoholic fatty liver disease, as proven by meta-analyses and clinical studies [1, 2, 15, 16]. A mean reduction of 0.25 BMI-SDS is similar to a reduction of 1 BMI or to a stable weight of over 1 year in growing children.

Even if RCTs and meta-analyses have proven a significant effect of obesity treatment programmes on BMI and cardiovascular risk factors in obese children, some concerns have to be mentioned. The obesity treatment trials were generally of small or moderate sample size, and the majority of the trials were of relatively short-term follow-up and included only a few children with a low social status or migration background [3]. Knowing these limitations, it is not surprising that RCTs likely overestimate the effectiveness of obesity treatment programmes in clinical practice [2].

Reasons for Failure of Obesity Treatment Programmes for Children and Adolescents

First, most overweight and obese children and their families do not want to participate in obesity treatment programmes [2]. Second, it can be speculated that the high dropout rate of clinical trials is caused by certain characteristics of obese patients and their families (e.g. lack of psychosocial support and parenting skills), by a decline in the motivation for lifestyle changes, by inadvertent constraints to therapy adherence, and by insufficient efficacy and/or quality of obesity treatment programmes or education of the therapists.

A factor contributing to weight regain may be the lack of a continued exercise programme, which fits well into a concept of obesity as a chronic disease [1]. The importance of exercise to sustain weight loss was concluded in several meta-analyses of long-term (3–5 years) weight maintenance studies in adults and children [13, 17].

Another important explanation for the difficulties in maintaining weight loss is the complex regulation of body weight. Body weight is centrally regulated, with peripheral hormonal signals released from the gastrointestinal tract, pancreas, and adipose tissue that regulate food intake and energy expenditure in the hypothalamus [2]. Many hormones, such as leptin, ghrelin, peptide YY, and insulin as well as others, have been found to influence appetite [2]. Furthermore, thyroid hormones determine the resting energy metabolic rate, but the underlying pathways are not fully understood [2, 18, 19]. In obese children, most of these hormones are altered as the adaption process increases the resting metabolic rate and increases satiety [2]. Weight loss results in acute compensatory changes in these hormones in obese adults and children, most of which reduce satiety and the resting metabolic rate and promote weight regain [2]. Accordingly, profound reductions in energy expenditures have been measured in obese humans who have lost weight [2]. In summary, multiple compensatory mechanisms that encourage weight gain must be overcome in order to maintain weight loss in obese children. Therefore, the high rate of relapse among obese children has a physiological basis and is not simply the result of lack of motivation.

Furthermore, the genetic background influences the outcome of obesity treatment programmes [2]. For example, a functionally relevant mutation in the melanocortin 4 receptor is associated with poorer outcome in obesity treatment programmes for children [20]. However, most single-nucleotide polymorphisms associated with obesity [21] are not related to weight loss in obesity treatment programmes or in subsequent weight regain [22]. Finally, children with metabolic syndrome respond to obesity intervention programmes to a lower degree, likely due to a background of insulin resistance [23].

In conclusion, blaming obese children and adolescents as well as their parents for unsuccessful weight loss seems inadequate due to the effects of different genetic and physiological backgrounds as well as to the multiple counter-regulations that occur to avoid weight loss.

Challenges of Obesity Treatment Programmes

Even if our knowledge concerning obesity treatment programmes in obese children is increasing, there are several unclear issues. We do not know the minimum amount of time and intensity that is needed for an obesity treatment programme. Contrary to the comprehensive literature on the effectiveness of these programmes, the literature on the cost-effectiveness of interventions that fight obesity in children is very limited [2]. The first studies reported that interventions to treat childhood obesity are potentially cost effective; however, the cost savings and health benefits may not appear until the sixth or seventh decade of life [2, 24].

We do not know what dietary advice and which components of exercise treatment are effective. It is clear that a special education of therapists is needed, but it is unclear which components are essential. Furthermore, since obesity is a chronic disease post-treatment, maintenance programmes are needed, but what should these programmes be composed of and how long are they needed? The greatest challenges are treatment of unmotivated obese children and adolescents, disabled obese children and adolescents, as well as extremely obese adolescents.

Conclusions

In summary, obesity treatment programmes are effective in reducing overweight in children if the parents are involved. Currently, a stable weight in growing children is associated with an improvement of cardiovascular risk factors and comorbidities of obesity. Failures in weight reduction are not only attributed to a lack of motivation and willingness to change behaviour but also to the genetic background and adaptive hormonal changes, which result in reduced resting metabolic rate and increased hunger.

The degree of weight loss due to obesity treatment programmes is only moderate. Furthermore, RCTs are likely to overestimate the effectiveness of interventions. However, we should not retreat into a state of therapeutic nihilism. Obesity treatment programmes should be primarily offered to children with successful change (such as young and less-overweight, motivated children), and we have to accept that lifestyle intervention is not effective for every obese child (particularly extremely obese adolescents). If obesity treatment programmes do not work, drug treatment of comorbidities and cardiovascular risk factors is necessary. There is still a great need for high-quality, multi-centre trials with long-term follow-up that are aimed to improve obesity treatment programmes.

This chapter was adapted from the publication 'Lifestyle intervention in childhood obesity: changes and challenges' by Thomas Reinehr in Nat Rev Endocrinol 2013;9:607–614.

References

1 August GP, Caprio S, Fennoy I, Freemark M, Kaufman FR, Lustig RH, Silverstein JH, Speiser PW, Styne DM, Montori VM: Prevention and treatment of pediatric obesity: an endocrine society clinical practice guideline based on expert opinion. J Clin Endocrinol Metab 2008;93:4576–4599.

2 Reinehr T: Lifestyle intervention in childhood obesity: changes and challenges. Nat Rev Endocrinol 2013;9:607–614.

3 Oude LH, Baur L, Jansen H, Shrewsbury VA, O'Malley C, Stolk RP, Summerbell CD: Interventions for treating obesity in children. Cochrane Database Syst Rev 2009;CD001872.

4 McGovern L, Johnson JN, Paulo R, Hettinger A, Singhal V, Kamath C, Erwin PJ, Montori VM: Clinical review: treatment of pediatric obesity: a systematic review and meta-analysis of randomized trials. J Clin Endocrinol Metab 2008;93:4600–4605.

5 Casazza K, Fontaine KR, Astrup A, Birch LL, Brown AW, Bohan Brown MM, Durant N, Dutton G, Foster EM, Heymsfield SB, McIver K, Mehta T, Menachemi N, Newby PK, Pate R, Rolls BJ, Sen B, Smith DL Jr, Thomas DM, Allison DB: Myths, presumptions, and facts about obesity. N Engl J Med 2013;368:446–454.

6 Skinner AC, Steiner MJ, Perrin EM: Self-reported energy intake by age in overweight and healthy-weight children in NHANES, 2001–2008. Pediatrics 2012;130:e936–e942.

7 Muckelbauer R, Libuda L, Clausen K, Toschke AM, Reinehr T, Kersting M: Promotion and provision of drinking water in schools for overweight prevention: randomized, controlled cluster trial. Pediatrics 2009;123:e661–e667.

8 Ebbeling CB, Feldman HA, Chomitz VR, Antonelli TA, Gortmaker SL, Osganian SK, Ludwig DS: A randomized trial of sugar-sweetened beverages and adolescent body weight. N Engl J Med 2012;367:1407–1416.

9 Wahi G, Parkin PC, Beyene J, Uleryk EM, Birken CS: Effectiveness of interventions aimed at reducing screen time in children: a systematic review and meta-analysis of randomized controlled trials. Arch Pediatr Adolesc Med 2011;165:979–986.

10 Epstein LH, Roemmich JN, Raynor HA: Behavioral therapy in the treatment of pediatric obesity. Pediatr Clin North Am 2001;48:981–993.

11 Sung-Chan P, Sung YW, Zhao X, Brownson RC: Family-based models for childhood-obesity intervention: a systematic review of randomized controlled trials. Obes Rev 2013;14:265–278.

12 Resnicow K, Davis R, Rollnick S: Motivational interviewing for pediatric obesity: conceptual issues and evidence review. J Am Diet Assoc 2006;106:2024–2033.

13 Anderson JW, Konz EC, Frederich RC, Wood CL: Long-term weight-loss maintenance: a meta-analysis of US studies. Am J Clin Nutr 2001;74:579–584.

14 Schaefer A, Winkel K, Finne E, Kolip P, Reinehr T: An effective lifestyle intervention in overweight children: one-year follow-up after the randomized controlled trial on 'Obeldicks light'. Clin Nutr 2011;30:629–633.

15 Ho M, Garnett SP, Baur L, Burrows T, Stewart L, Neve M, Collins C: Effectiveness of lifestyle interventions in child obesity: systematic review with meta-analysis. Pediatrics 2012;130:e1647–e1671.

16 Ford AL, Hunt LP, Cooper A, Shield JP: What reduction in BMI SDS is required in obese adolescents to improve body composition and cardiometabolic health? Arch Dis Child 2010;95:256–261.

17 Wilfley DE, Stein RI, Saelens BE, Mockus DS, Matt GE, Hayden-Wade HA, Welch RR, Schechtman KB, Thompson PA, Epstein LH: Efficacy of maintenance treatment approaches for childhood overweight: a randomized controlled trial. JAMA 2007;298:1661–1673.

18 Reinehr T: Obesity and thyroid function. Mol Cell Endocrinol 2010;316:165–171.

19 Wolters B, Lass N, Reinehr T: Thyrotropin and free triiodothyronine concentrations are associated to weight loss in lifestyle intervention and weight regain afterwards in obese children. Eur J Endocrinol 2013;168:323–329.

20 Reinehr T, Hebebrand J, Friedel S, Toschke AM, Brumm H, Biebermann H, Hinney A: Lifestyle intervention in obese children with variations in the melanocortin 4 receptor gene. Obesity (Silver Spring) 2009;17:382–389.

21 Speliotes EK, Willer CJ, Berndt SI, Monda KL, Thorleifsson G, Jackson AU, Allen HL, Lindgren CM, Luan J, Magi R, Randall JC, Vedantam S, Winkler TW, Qi L, Workalemahu T, Heid IM, Steinthorsdottir V, Stringham HM, Weedon MN, Wheeler E, Wood AR, Ferreira T, Weyant RJ, Segre AV, Estrada K, Liang L, Nemesh J, Park JH, Gustafsson S, Kilpelainen TO, Yang J, Bouatia-Naji N, Esko T, Feitosa MF, Kutalik Z, Mangino M, Raychaudhuri S, Scherag A, Smith AV, Welch R, Zhao JH, Aben KK, Absher DM, Amin N, Dixon AL, Fisher E, Glazer NL, Goddard ME, Heard-Costa NL, Hoesel V, Hottenga JJ, Johansson A, Johnson T, Ketkar S, Lamina C, Li S,

Moffatt MF, Myers RH, Narisu N, Perry JR, Peters MJ, Preuss M, Ripatti S, Rivadeneira F, Sandholt C, Scott LJ, Timpson NJ, Tyrer JP, van WS, Watanabe RM, White CC, Wiklund F, Barlassina C, Chasman DI, Cooper MN, Jansson JO, Lawrence RW, Pellikka N, Prokopenko I, Shi J, Thiering E, Alavere H, Alibrandi MT, Almgren P, Arnold AM, Aspelund T, Atwood LD, Balkau B, Balmforth AJ, Bennett AJ, Ben-Shlomo Y, Bergman RN, Bergmann S, Biebermann H, Blakemore AI, Boes T, Bonnycastle LL, Bornstein SR, Brown MJ, Buchanan TA, Busonero F, Campbell H, Cappuccio FP, Cavalcanti-Proenca C, Chen YD, Chen CM, Chines PS, Clarke R, Coin L, Connell J, Day IN, Heijer M, Duan J, Ebrahim S, Elliott P, Elosua R, Eiriksdottir G, Erdos MR, Eriksson JG, Facheris MF, Felix SB, Fischer-Posovszky P, Folsom AR, Friedrich N, Freimer NB, Fu M, Gaget S, Gejman PV, Geus EJ, Gieger C, Gjesing AP, Goel A, Goyette P, Grallert H, Grassler J, Greenawalt DM, Groves CJ, Gudnason V, Guiducci C, Hartikainen AL, Hassanali N, Hall AS, Havulinna AS, Hayward C, Heath AC, Hengstenberg C, Hicks AA, Hinney A, Hofman A, Homuth G, Hui J, Igl W, Iribarren C, Isomaa B, Jacobs KB, Jarick I, Jewell E, John U, Jorgensen T, Jousilahti P, Jula A, Kaakinen M, Kajantie E, Kaplan LM, Kathiresan S, Kettunen J, Kinnunen L, Knowles JW, Kolcic I, Konig IR, Koskinen S, Kovacs P, Kuusisto J, Kraft P, Kvaloy K, Laitinen J, Lantieri O, Lanzani C, Launer LJ, Lecoeur C, Lehtimaki T, Lettre G, Liu J, Lokki ML, Lorentzon M, Luben RN, Ludwig B, Manunta P, Marek D, Marre M, Martin NG, McArdle WL, McCarthy A, McKnight B, Meitinger T, Melander O, Meyre D, Midthjell K, Montgomery GW, Morken MA, Morris AP, Mulic R, Ngwa JS, Nelis M, Neville MJ, Nyholt DR, O'Donnell CJ, O'Rahilly S, Ong KK, Oostra B, Pare G, Parker AN, Perola M, Pichler I, Pietilainen KH, Platou CG, Polasek O, Pouta A, Rafelt S, Raitakari O, Rayner NW, Ridderstrale M, Rief W, Ruokonen A, Robertson NR, Rzehak P, Salomaa V, Sanders AR, Sandhu MS, Sanna S, Saramies J, Savolainen MJ, Scherag S, Schipf S, Schreiber S, Schunkert H, Silander K, Sinisalo J, Siscovick DS, Smit JH, Soranzo N, Sovio U, Stephens J, Surakka I, Swift AJ, Tammesoo ML, Tardif JC, Teder-Laving M, Teslovich TM, Thompson JR, Thomson B, Tonjes A, Tuomi T, van Meurs JB, van Ommen GJ: Association analyses of 249,796 individuals reveal 18 new loci associated with body mass index. Nat Genet 2010;42:937–948.

22 Hinney A, Wolters B, Putter C, Grallert H, Illig T, Hebebrand J, Reinehr T: No impact of obesity susceptibility loci on weight regain after a lifestyle intervention in overweight children. J Pediatr Endocrinol Metab 2013;26:1209–1213.

23 Uysal Y, Wolters B, Knop CRT: Components of the metabolic syndrome are negative predictors of weight loss in obese children with lifestyle intervention. Clin Nutr 2014;33:620–625.

24 Hollingworth W, Hawkins J, Lawlor DA, Brown M, Marsh T, Kipping RR: Economic evaluation of lifestyle interventions to treat overweight or obesity in children. Int J Obes (Lond) 2012;36:559–566.

Prof. Dr. Thomas Reinehr
Department of Paediatric Endocrinology, Diabetes and Nutrition Medicine
Vestische Hospital for Children and Adolescents, University of Witten/Herdecke
Dr. F. Steiner Strasse 5
DE–45711 Datteln (Germany)
E-Mail T.Reinehr@kinderklinik-datteln.de

Kiess W, Wabitsch M, Maffeis C, Sharma AM (eds): Metabolic Syndrome and Obesity in Childhood and Adolescence.
Pediatr Adolesc Med. Basel, Karger, 2015, vol 19, pp 179–186 (DOI: 10.1159/000368135)

Adolescent Bariatric Surgery: Current Status in an Evolving Field

Paola Luca[a] · Elizabeth Dettmer[b] · Jacob C. Langer[c] · Jill K. Hamilton[d]

[a]Section of Endocrinology, Alberta Children's Hospital, Calgary, Alb., [b]Department of Psychology, [c]Division of General and Thoracic Surgery, and [d]Division of Endocrinology, The Hospital for Sick Children, Toronto, Ont., Canada

Abstract

Bariatric surgery has been increasingly performed in adolescents over the past decade. Consensus guidelines have been developed to help heath care teams select adolescent candidates for surgery. Reports of short-term outcomes in adolescents have demonstrated similar BMI reduction and safety as in the adult population. There are several issues specific to adolescents that require further consideration, including a lower age limit and BMI at surgery, the optimal choice of bariatric procedure, the potential for the development of disordered eating and weight recidivism after surgery, and the extent of psychological and developmental assessment prior to performing these procedures. With the ongoing increase in the number of adolescent bariatric surgeries performed, it will be essential for high-level evidence with long-term follow-up to be generated to help address these issues and guide health care teams caring for teens with obesity.

Overview of Adolescent Bariatric Surgery

Bariatric surgery was first performed in adolescents beginning in the late 1970s, and the number of procedures performed has progressively increased over time. Data from the Kids' Inpatient Database [1] suggest that the number of bariatric operations in children and adolescents in the U.S. has doubled from 771 in 2003 to 1,615 in 2009. The increase is likely due to increasing rates of adult bariatric surgery and the knowledge that nonsurgical treatments have a limited effect on children with severe obesity and that, without an effective intervention, the majority of obese adolescents will remain obese in adulthood [2].

The most common types of bariatric operations performed in adolescents include Roux-en-Y gastric bypass (RYGB), laparoscopic adjustable gastric banding (LAGB), and sleeve gastrectomy (SG) (fig. 1) [3]. RYGB is both a restrictive and a

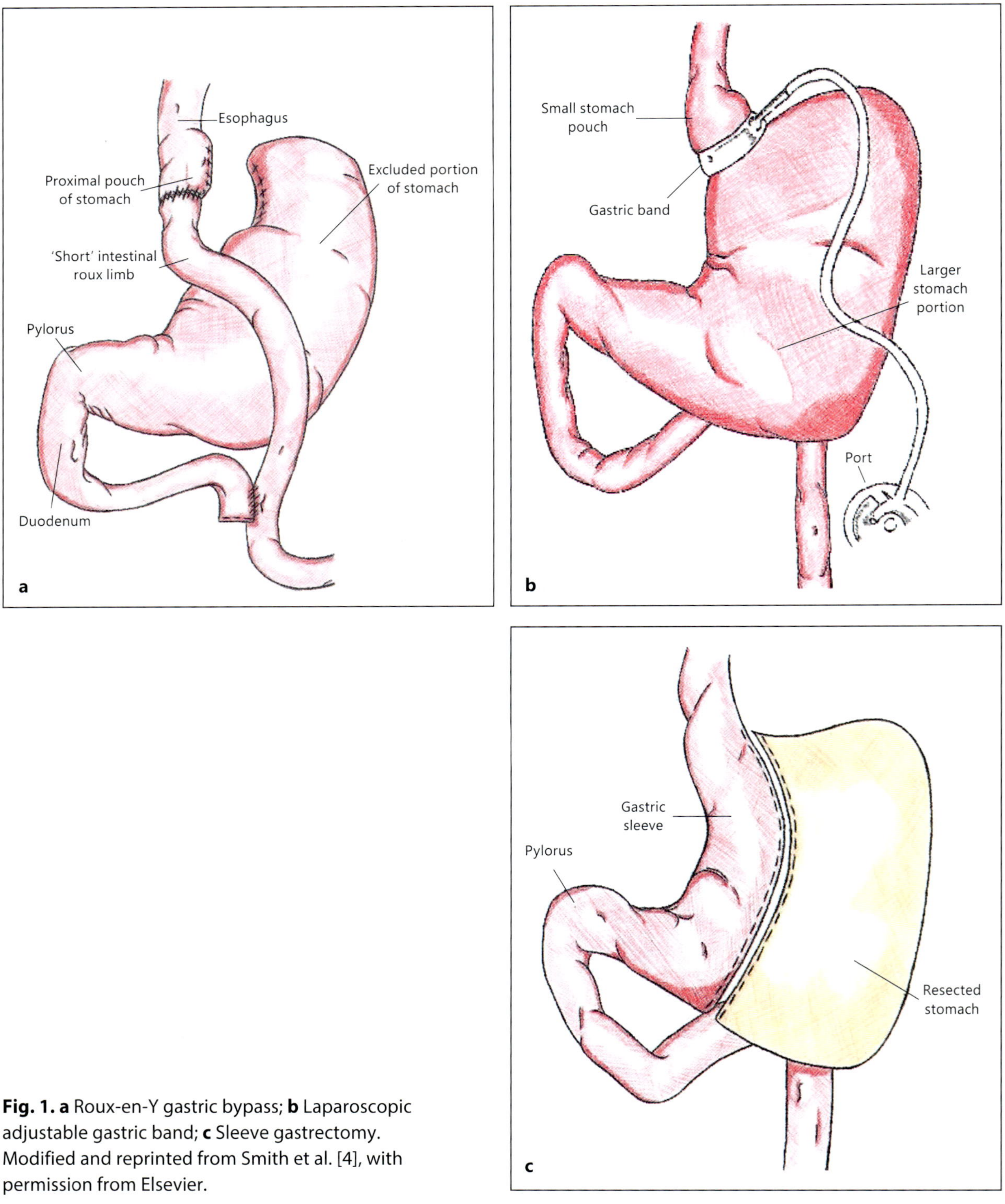

Fig. 1. a Roux-en-Y gastric bypass; **b** Laparoscopic adjustable gastric band; **c** Sleeve gastrectomy. Modified and reprinted from Smith et al. [4], with permission from Elsevier.

malabsorptive procedure that involves creating a small gastric pouch below the gastroesophageal junction and connecting a Roux-en-Y limb of the jejunum to the pouch [4]. LAGB is a purely restrictive operation in which a band is placed around the proximal aspect of the stomach, below the gastroesophageal junction. Additionally, a catheter attached to the band is connected to an infusion port placed on the abdominal wall for saline injection to tighten or loosen the band [4]. SG is a relatively new procedure in both adults and adolescents. It is a restrictive procedure in which most of the stomach is removed, leaving a tabularized stomach along the lesser curve that is 85–90% smaller than its original size [4, 5]. All three operations are done laparoscopically in almost all cases. Due to concern about long-term nutrient deficiencies associated with malabsorptive procedures as well as lower long-term weight loss with LAGB, SG is often recommended for adolescent patients [6].

Patient Selection

Recently, the American Society for Metabolic and Bariatric Surgery Pediatric Committee [3] published best-practice guidelines on adolescent bariatric surgery. Patient criteria include adolescents with a BMI $\geq$35 kg/m^2 and with major co-morbidities, including type 2 diabetes mellitus (T2DM), moderate to severe sleep apnea, pseudotumor cerebri, or severe nonalcoholic steatohepatitis, or with a BMI $\geq$40 kg/m^2 and with other co-morbidities (e.g. hypertension, glucose intolerance, dyslipidemia) [3]. Adolescents should be postpubertal, have completed at least 95% of their estimated growth if undergoing a diversional or malabsorptive procedure, and have demonstrated an understanding of the lifestyle changes needed after surgery [7]. In addition, a psychosocial assessment should demonstrate that the adolescent is capable of making an informed decision and is aware of the risks and benefits of surgery; that the teen has social support; and that, together with his/her family, the teen is able to adhere to pre- and postoperative recommendations [7]. If the adolescent has a psychiatric condition such as depression or an eating disorder, it should be treated and stabilized prior to pursuing bariatric surgery [7]. All operations should be performed in specialized bariatric centers [7].

Outcomes after Adolescent Bariatric Surgery

Knowledge of outcomes after adolescent bariatric surgery is increasing but is still limited due to the retrospective nature of the majority of studies, heterogeneity among studies, and the small sample sizes and short follow-up times of studies [5]. A meta-analysis of bariatric surgery in 637 pediatric patients showed an average weighted mean BMI difference from baseline to 1 year of –13.5 kg/m^2 [5]. When analyzed by surgery type, RYGB was associated with an average BMI loss at 12 months of −17.2 kg/m^2, in contrast to −10.5 kg/m^2 for LAGB [5]. For SG, the mean BMI loss was intermediate, or −14.5 kg/m^2, based on three studies [5]. Since the publication of the meta-analysis, prospective studies from Germany, the U.S., and Canada have shown comparable outcomes [6, 8, 9]. These results are also quite comparable with those in the adult population, with an average BMI reduction of −14.2 kg/m^2 reported in a meta-analysis [10].

Although long-term safety data are still lacking, shorter-term information is available. The Teen-Longitudinal Assessment of Bariatric Surgery [11] study reported on the perioperative outcomes of 242 adolescents aged 19 years or younger who underwent bariatric surgery in the U.S. from 2007 to 2011. This was the first study to prospectively collect standardized data from multiple centers performing bariatric surgery, whereas other studies have used registry-based data, which can be prone to incomplete data and coding errors [8, 11]. The average age was 17.1 years among the patients, who had a median BMI of 50.5 kg/m^2, and 51% had ≥4 major co-morbidities [11]. Overall, within 30 days of surgery, 19 patients (8%) experienced a major complication, and 36 (15%) had a minor complication [11]. There were no reported deaths within 30 days of the procedure [11]. The majority of complications took place before discharge from the hospital: 5% had a major perioperative complication, including 7 patients who underwent reoperation for bowel obstruction/bleeding, gastrointestinal (GI) leak/sepsis, or suspected sepsis; 4 patients who required a transfusion for postoperative bleeding; one patient who required anticoagulation for deep venous thrombosis; and one patient who had a splenectomy after intraoperative splenic injury [11]. In total, 8% had a minor perioperative complication, with urinary tract events being the most common [11]. After discharge and within 30 days of surgery, 3% had a major complication (pulmonary embolus or GI leak), and 11% had a minor complication (anastomotic stricture; wound infection; or GI symptoms, such as abdominal pain and nausea) [11]. In a study comparing outcomes between adults and adolescents undergoing bariatric surgery in the U.S. between 2002 and 2006, adolescents demonstrated a lower 30-day complication rate (5.5%) compared with adults (9.8%), with similarly low rates of in-hospital mortality (no adolescent deaths vs 0.2% in adults) [12].

Bariatric surgery performed in adolescents results in rapid improvement of obesity-related comorbidities. A German registry study reported that rates of diabetes, hypertension, and sleep apnea were reduced by approximately half in 167 adolescents and young adults following gastric bypass, LAGB, or SG at 18 months of follow-up [8]. In a report on adolescents with T2DM who underwent RYGB 1 year postoperatively, 10 of 11 patients no longer required oral medication, and one patient remained on insulin, but at a much lower dose, without additional oral therapy [13]. Surgery was also associated with significant improvements in BMI, hemoglobin A1C levels, lipid levels, and blood pressure [13]. Finally, the largest report on outcomes after SG, performed in Saudi Arabia among 108 children and adolescents (aged 5–21 years old), found that patients with available data demonstrated resolution rates of 70% for dyslipidemia, 75% for hypertension, 94% for diabetes, 100% for prediabetes, and 91% for symptoms of sleep apnea [14].

The impact of bariatric surgery on psychosocial functioning is less well known. Two-year data after RYGB in 16 adolescents showed weight reduction, improved health-related quality of life and self-concept, and a decrease in depressive symptoms across the first year postsurgery and decelerations in the second year, accompanied by weight regain, slight increases in depressive symptoms, and decreases in health-related quality of life and self-concept [15]. A short-term study from Sweden in 37 adolescents 4 months after RYGB demonstrated an overall significant improvement in symptoms of anxiety, depression, and self-concept from baseline and no significant change in anger or disruptive behavior. However, 16% of adolescents exhibited deterioration in two or more of these aspects, suggesting the need for close psychological monitoring after bariatric surgery [16]. Adolescence is a complex developmental stage during which self-identity is developing and a sense of belonging is central. Rapid changes in BMI and related increases in social acceptance or unexpected continued marginalization can lead to complicated positive or negative psychological sequelae, respectively, that need to be better understood.

Controversies in Adolescent Bariatric Surgery

While the amount of data on adolescent bariatric surgery is growing, the acceptability of this procedure in children and adolescents continues to be a controversial topic [17]. Further research is needed to identify which specific procedure is optimal for adolescents, who should be operated on, who should be operating, how patients should be followed up, and the optimal timing of surgery that provides the largest benefit-to-harm ratio [5, 17]. Despite this, there are currently reports of children as young as 2 $^1/_2$ years of age undergoing irreversible bariatric surgery [18]. Another debated topic is whether surgery should occur at lower BMIs. Studies from North America and Europe have demonstrated that preoperative BMI is an accurate indicator of nadir BMI at 1–2 years post-bariatric surgery, with a 1/3 reduction in BMI from the preoperative BMI, suggesting that referral at a later stage or higher BMI may prevent attainment of a nonobese BMI [19, 20]. In adults, the criteria for bariatric surgery now include a BMI of 30–34.9 kg/m^2 and T2DM or metabolic syndrome, although there currently is limited evidence to support this decision [21]. Whether the adult trends will translate into lower BMI criteria for adolescents remains to be seen.

A challenging ethical issue is the ability to obtain valid informed consent from the adolescent and his/her family. The adolescent's capacity to make this decision requires assessment, and informed assent/consent should be obtained separately from the parents to avoid coercion [7, 22]. Parents may feel responsible and guilty for their child's obesity, which may influence their attitude toward surgery [17]. It is also very important that adolescents and families understand that bariatric surgery is not a 'quick fix', but rather a tool to help them with ongoing healthy behavioral changes, and that a lack of adherence to recommended eating advice will ultimately lead to weight regain. Adolescents' decisions may also be driven by the belief that achieving a certain thinness will impart happiness and success, and this may impede their full appreciation of the risks of surgery. For these reasons, it is recommended that the process of obtaining consent for surgery take place over several months, while families participate in behavioral modification programs [6, 22]. Discussions should include the different surgical options, the risks and benefit of each procedure, the likely outcomes, and the uncertainty of long-term outcomes in adolescents [22].

There are particular negative sequelae of bariatric surgery reported in adult studies that may be of greater concern in the adolescent. The first is the impact of bariatric surgery on the development of disordered eating in adolescents, especially since these symptoms are often present prior to surgery. For example, an assessment of 200 adolescents prior to surgery demonstrated that 4% met the criteria for an eating disorder, 16% reported current binge eating, 9.5% reported current night eating, and 1% were purging [23]. Another negative consequence of bariatric surgery in adults is the presence of excess skin following major weight loss [24], which in our experience, can be of particular concern to the adolescent. Many adolescents seeking bariatric surgery have experienced a long history of social isolation, bullying, and a lack of intimate relationships [25]. With rapid weight loss, changes in self-esteem and body image and increased fertility may leave females particularly vulnerable to an increase in unwanted pregnancy [26]. As such, adolescent females who undergo bariatric surgery require counseling in regards to their reproductive health now and in the future [27], and some groups advocate insertion of a contraceptive intrauterine device at the time of the bariatric procedure [26].

Weight recidivism in adults post-bariatric surgery is reported to occur in up to 80% of patients. However, the majority remain significantly below their presurgery weight, with only 10–20% regaining a significant proportion of their excess weight [28]. After RYGB, weight regain varied between 10 and 15% among adolescent patients in two small studies after 6–12 years, similar to reports of weight regain in adults after gastric bypass [29, 30].

As bariatric surgery becomes a more accepted form of treatment for adolescents with severe obesity, equitable access to this treatment is an important ethical consideration. In adults, disparities in access to bariatric surgery were found in the U.S., with fewer African Americans, Hispanics, low-income individuals, and males undergoing surgery than would be expected [31]. Similar data are not yet available for children and adolescents. However, a survey of pediatricians and family doctors revealed that nearly 1/2 of physicians would never refer an obese adolescent for bariatric surgery, and a similar proportion felt that the minimum age for a referral should be 18 years [32]. The reason for this hesitation is not known but may be due to unfamiliarity with the procedure and concern about the decision-making capacity of adolescents [32]. It is quite likely that many severely obese adolescents desiring bariatric surgery are not referred based on the opinion of their primary care physician.

In summary, adolescent bariatric surgery is an effective treatment option for select patients when other interventions have failed. Prospective data are emerging on the outcomes and complications of bariatric procedures, although there remain many unanswered questions and several areas of consideration unique to the developmental phase of adolescence. The ongoing generation of high-quality evidence is required to address these issues and should assist practitioners in managing the ethical and controversial issues that accompany bariatric surgery in adolescents.

References

1 Zwintscher NP, Azarow KS, Horton JD, et al: The increasing incidence of adolescent bariatric surgery. J Pediatr Surg 2013;48:2401–2407.
2 Treadwell JR, Sun F, Schoelles K: Systematic review and meta-analysis of bariatric surgery for pediatric obesity. Ann Surg 2008;248:763–776.
3 Michalsky M, Reichard K, Inge T, et al: ASMBS Pediatric Committee best practice guidelines. Surg Obes Relat Dis 2012;8:1–7.
4 Smith BR, Schauer P, Nguyen NT: Surgical approaches to the treatment of obesity: bariatric surgery. Endocrinol Metab Clin North Am 2008;37: 943–964.
5 Black JA, White B, Viner RM, et al: Bariatric surgery for obese children and adolescents: a systematic review and meta-analysis. Obes Rev 2013;14:634–644.
6 Davies DA, Hamilton J, Dettmer E, et al: Adolescent bariatric surgery: the Canadian perspective. Semin Pediatr Surg 2014;23:31–36.
7 Pratt JS, Lenders CM, Dionne EA, et al: Best practice updates for pediatric/adolescent weight loss surgery. Obesity (Silver Spring) 2009;17:901–910.
8 Lennerz BS, Wabitsch M, Lippert H, et al: Bariatric surgery in adolescents and young adults-safety and effectiveness in a cohort of 345 patients. Int J Obes 2005;2014:334–340.
9 Messiah SE, Lopez-Mitnik G, Winegar D, et al: Changes in weight and co-morbidities among adolescents undergoing bariatric surgery: 1-year results from the Bariatric Outcomes Longitudinal Database. Surg Obes Relat Dis 2013;9:503–513.
10 Buchwald H, Avidor Y, Braunwald E, et al: Bariatric surgery: a systematic review and meta-analysis. JAMA 2004;292:1724–1737.
11 Inge TH, Zeller MH, Jenkins TM, et al: Perioperative outcomes of adolescents undergoing bariatric surgery: the Teen-Longitudinal Assessment Of Bariatric Surgery (Teen-LABS) study. JAMA Pediatr 2014; 168:47–53.
12 Varela JE, Hinojosa MW, Nguyen NT: Perioperative outcomes of bariatric surgery in adolescents compared with adults at academic medical centers. Surg Obes Relat Dis 2007;3:537–540, discussion: 541–542.
13 Inge TH, Miyano G, Bean J, et al: Reversal of type 2 diabetes mellitus and improvements in cardiovascular risk factors after surgical weight loss in adolescents. Pediatrics 2009;123:214–222.
14 Alqahtani AR, Antonisamy B, Alamri H, et al: Laparoscopic sleeve gastrectomy in 108 obese children and adolescents aged 5 to 21 years. Ann Surg 2012; 256:266–273.
15 Zeller MH, Reiter-Purtill J, Ratcliff MB, et al: Two-year trends in psychosocial functioning after adolescent roux-en-Y gastric bypass. Surg Obes Relat Dis 2011;7:727–732.
16 Jarvholm K, Olbers T, Marcus C, et al: Short-term psychological outcomes in severely obese adolescents after bariatric surgery. Obesity (Silver Spring, MD) 2012;20:318–323.
17 Hofmann B: Bariatric surgery for obese children and adolescents: a review of the moral challenges. BMC Med Ethics 2013;14:18.
18 Mohaidly MA, Suliman A, Malawi H: Laparoscopic sleeve gastrectomy for a two-and half year old morbidly obese child. Int J Surg Case Rep 2013;4:1057–1060.
19 Inge TH, Jenkins TM, Zeller M, et al: Baseline BMI is a strong predictor of nadir BMI after adolescent gastric bypass. J Pediatr 2010;156:103–108.e1.
20 Olbers T, Gronowitz E, Werling M, et al: Two-year outcome of laparoscopic roux-en-Y gastric bypass in adolescents with severe obesity: results from a Swedish Nationwide Study (AMOS). Int J Obes 2005; 2012:1388–1395.

21 Mechanick JI, Youdim A, Jones DB, et al: Clinical practice guidelines for the perioperative nutritional, metabolic, and nonsurgical support of the bariatric surgery patient – 2013 update: cosponsored by American Association of Clinical Endocrinologists, the Obesity Society, and American Society for Metabolic & Bariatric Surgery. Endocr Pract 2013;19:337–372.
22 Caniano DA: Ethical issues in pediatric bariatric surgery. Semin Pediatr Surg 2009;18:186–192.
23 Sysko R, Zandberg LJ, Devlin MJ, et al: Mental health evaluations for adolescents Prior to bariatric surgery: a review of existing practices and a specific example of assessment procedures. Clinical Obesity 2013;3:62–72.
24 Steffen KJ, Sarwer DB, Thompson JK, et al: Predictors of satisfaction with excess skin and desire for body contouring after bariatric surgery. Surg Obes Relat Dis 2012;8:92–97.
25 Cheng YH, Landale NS: Adolescent overweight, social relationships and the transition to first sex: gender and racial variations. Perspect Sex Reprod Health 2011;43:6–15.
26 Hillman JB, Miller RJ, Inge TH: Menstrual concerns and intrauterine contraception among adolescent bariatric surgery patients. J Womens Health 2002; 2011:533–538.
27 Roehrig HR, Xanthakos SA, Sweeney J, et al: Pregnancy after gastric bypass surgery in adolescents. Obes Surg 2007;17:873–877.
28 Karmali S, Brar B, Shi X, et al: Weight recidivism post-bariatric surgery: a systematic review. Obes Surg 2013;23:1922–1933.
29 Strauss RS, Bradley LJ, Brolin RE: Gastric bypass surgery in adolescents with morbid obesity. J Pediatr 2001;138:499–504.
30 Rand CS, Macgregor AM: Adolescents having obesity surgery: a 6-year follow-up. South Med J 1994; 87:1208–1213.
31 Flum DR, Khan TV, Dellinger EP: Toward the rational and equitable use of bariatric surgery. JAMA 2007;298:1442–1444.
32 Woolford SJ, Clark SJ, Gebremariam A, et al: To cut or not to cut: physicians' perspectives on referring adolescents for bariatric surgery. Obes Surg 2010;20: 937–942.

Jill K. Hamilton, MD, MSc, FRCPC
Division of Endocrinology, The Hospital for Sick Children
555 University Avenue
Toronto, ON, M5G 1X8 (Canada)
E-Mail jill.hamilton@sickkids.ca

Kiess W, Wabitsch M, Maffeis C, Sharma AM (eds): Metabolic Syndrome and Obesity in Childhood and Adolescence. Pediatr Adolesc Med. Basel, Karger, 2015, vol 19, pp 187–193 (DOI: 10.1159/000368136)

Beyond Weight Loss: Experiences and Insights Related to Working Effectively with Families and Operating within the Health Care System to Manage Pediatric Obesity

Geoff D.C. Ball[a, b] · Jillian L.S. Avis[a] · Annick Buchholz[c] · Tracey Bridger[d, e] · Jean-Pierre Chanoine[f] · Stasia Hadjiyannakis[c] · Jill K. Hamilton[g] · Laurent Legault[h] · Katherine M. Morrison[i] · Anne Wareham[e] · Mary M. Jetha[a, b]

[a]Department of Pediatrics, Faculty of Medicine and Dentistry, University of Alberta, Edmonton, Alta., [b]Pediatric Centre for Weight and Health, Stollery Children's Hospital, Alberta Health Services, Edmonton, Alta., [c]The Children's Hospital of Eastern Ontario (CHEO) Research Institute, Ottawa, Ont., [d]Department of Pediatrics, Faculty of Medicine, Memorial University, St. John's, Nfld., [e]Janeway Children's Health and Rehabilitation Centre, St. John's, Nfld., [f]Endocrinology and Diabetes Unit, Department of Pediatrics, University of British Columbia, Vancouver, B.C., and British Columbia's Children's Hospital, Vancouver, B.C., [g]Division of Endocrinology, The Hospital for Sick Children, and Department of Pediatrics, University of Toronto, Toronto, Ont., [h]Department of Pediatrics, McGill University, Montreal, Que., and Montreal Children's Hospital, Montreal, Que., and [i]Department of Pediatrics, McMaster University, Hamilton, Ont., and McMaster Children's Hospital, Hamilton, Ont., Canada

Abstract

Pediatric obesity is an urgent and complex public health issue. The high proportions of children who meet the definition of overweight or obesity highlight the need for effective and accessible services to reduce short- and long-term health risks. In our experience, we have encountered a number of challenges common in pediatric obesity management across our clinical and research centers. For the purpose of this review, these challenges and our real-world experiences are grouped as issues that include (i) caring for children with obesity and their families and (ii) working within the health care system. Overall, we highlight a number of lessons learned from our years of experience and detail ongoing initiatives designed to optimize health services for managing obesity developed for children and their families.

Introduction

For clinicians working on the front line in the field of pediatric obesity, it can be discouraging that there is no single proven strategy for success in pediatric weight management. It is problematic even to define *success*, although most researchers, clinicians, funding agencies, government officials, and families would view weight loss as the most meaningful measure of success. However, as we continue to provide care for children with obesity and their families, we have become increasingly aware of the many complex issues that are involved in pediatric weight management and how these issues impact our ability to provide the best possible health services for managing obesity.

This chapter includes a brief review of key issues in providing obesity-related health services for children with obesity and their families. We have organized these issues into two broad categories: (i) caring for children with obesity and their families and (ii) working within the health care system. In regards to the former, we give special attention to providing family-centered care (FCC), tailoring health services, and addressing mental health in the population of interest. In relation to the health care system, we highlight the establishment of services for pediatric obesity management, the development of practical clinical resources and tools, and the common barriers experienced by families when accessing health services.

Caring for Children and Families

Family-centered Care: Managing pediatric obesity is most likely to be effective when strategies focus on healthy lifestyle changes within the family. FCC is based on mutually beneficial partnerships between health care professionals and family members during the planning, delivery, and evaluation of clinical care [1]. The family is empowered to adopt an active participating role in the child's care, and the clinicians adopt a collaborative role, which enhances the development of a constructive relationship between clinicians and families [1]. In this model, multiple family members have the potential to benefit from healthy changes [2], and it is equally important for the clinicians to gain respect and trust from the child. Clinicians can demonstrate FCC when discussing sensitive issues such as weight and lifestyle habits. Clinicians must provide a safe environment for communication in a nonjudgmental and unbiased manner, such as by using language that parents prefer when discussing children's weight status [3]. Caregivers should focus on families' successes, progress, and positive changes. Children's developmental maturity should be taken into account to best meet the needs of both younger children and adolescents, whose autonomy and dependency may differ.

Tailoring Health Services: Treatment plans should be tailored to children's and families' individual priorities and concerns. Clinical practice guidelines recommend that clinicians help families to identify modifiable barriers impacting weight management [4]. Each family comes from a unique environment and set of experiences that form their context for weight management. FCC allows the clinician to assess and consider weight management in each family according to that family's needs and priorities. Goals and strategies can be developed specifically in accordance with the capacity for and motivation to change and families' unique accessibility to resources and facilities. In addition, it is equally important to distinguish between children's challenges, strengths, and abilities and those of their parents. Treating each family member as unique also stems from FCC, promoting therapeutic alliances both with the child as an individual and with the family as a unit. The establishment of a strong alliance can positively influence families' engagement, reduce the likelihood that families will discontinue care prematurely, and increase the chances of treatment success [5].

The definition of success may vary between clinicians and families; however, more often than not, success is defined according to weight loss. In our experience, we have found that given the multifaceted nature of childhood obesity, which often also includes family obesity, it may be more appropriate to frame success in non-weight-related terms. For example, success may include positive health behavior change (e.g., more frequent healthy food choices); change in attitude (e.g., acceptance of the long-term nature of weight management); and/or improvements in relationships (e.g., between family members), psychosocial health (e.g., improved self-esteem), and/or metabolic markers (e.g., blood pressure). When clinicians and families agree on similar measures of non-weight-related success, stronger collaboration can be formed, and families may be more likely to continue with the program.

Mental Health: To date, an extensive amount of research has focused on the cardiometabolic risk associated with childhood obesity [6]; however, psychosocial issues are often more salient for families on a day-to-day basis. Internalizing (e.g., anxiety) and externalizing (e.g., hyperactivity) disorders and behaviors are common in children with obesity [7] and can complicate the implementation of and adherence to management strategies. These conditions may require assessment and treatment by a mental health professional (e.g., psychologist), and the importance of a mental health care provider as part of the weight management team cannot be understated.

Readiness to change is another essential consideration. Motivational variables (e.g., readiness, importance, confidence) vary among family members, vary with time, and differ according to the health behavior being addressed. If clinicians misinterpret or misjudge families' readiness to change, it is possible that the children and families will experience unnecessary barriers to successful weight management. Clinicians can acquire skills and techniques in motivational interviewing [8] and cognitive behavioral therapy [9] and incorporate these into practice. Mental health professionals can assist in the psychosocial, emotional, and cognitive aspects of weight management by (i) assuming leadership roles, (ii) providing direct support for families, and (iii) building pediatric mental health knowledge and skills among team members from other disciplines. Taken together, these realities highlight the need for mental health assessment and treatment as part of effective pediatric weight management.

Weight Bias: Negative attitudes and beliefs about an individual's body weight represent other factors that can negatively impact mental and emotional health and success in weight management. Many children and families in our care have experienced shame, blame, and stigmatization from other family members and from friends, teachers, co-workers, health professionals, and the media regarding the children's weight status. Unfortunately, weight bias is also common within health care and among professionals [10]. Stigmatizing and blaming attitudes from health care professionals undermine all aspects of FCC, as bias may hinder the establishment of mutual trust and an alliance between clinicians and families. Additionally, when children present with adverse psychosocial conditions (e.g., depression, low self-esteem), weight bias encountered in the health care setting may lead to decreased willingness to engage, an increased risk of worsening health, an increased need for health care, and perpetuation of this cycle [10]. In health care and in society, there is a clear need to shift from a focus on physical weight to a nonjudgmental and unbiased appreciation of the complex causes and consequences of obesity.

Working within the Health Care System

Establishing Health Services for Managing Pediatric Obesity: We work within a national universal health care system in Canada, although funding decisions for health services and the allocation of resources are made by provincial, regional, and local authorities. The high prevalence of obesity and its co-morbidities and the dissemination of this reality throughout society have highlighted the need for effective services. However, a number of challenges currently exist within Canadian programs, including relatively small numbers of referrals for weight management, failure of families to engage in treatment programs, high levels of attrition, and a lack of substantial weight loss for most children with obesity. Ongoing education, contextualization, and justification among colleagues and administrators within the health care system are essential for obesity to be viewed as a chronic condition that requires ongoing support and management. Framing obesity as a complex, chronic medical condition that requires extensive, multidisciplinary, and long-term health services would help to establish pediatric obesity as a legitimate pediatric subspecialty and to distinguish it from other specialty areas in pediatrics that provide high-intensity/short-term, low-intensity/short-term, or low-intensity/long-term treatments.

Two common issues that we have encountered in our health care environment are (i) a desire for practical clinical resources and tools that clinicians can use with families and (ii) the need to enhance the accessibility of health services, particularly for families living in remote or rural regions.

Practical Clinical Resources: Primary care clinicians desire practice-based tools to support families in managing pediatric obesity [11, 12]. In response, and complementary to a number of existing resources (e.g., Canada's Food Guide to Healthy Eating [13], Canadian Physical Activity Guidelines/Canadian Sedentary Behaviour Guidelines [14], World Health Organization Growth Reference [15]), team members have recently developed three *made-in-Canada* tools. First, the Edmonton Obesity Staging System for Pediatrics (EOSS-P), based on the original EOSS for adults [16], provides a comprehensive assessment of the health and well-being of children with obesity, beyond anthropometric data [17]. The EOSS-P is based on simple clinical assessments of *metabolic, mechanical, and mental health* and diagnostic evaluations that are available and routine in clinical practice. In addition, a measure of *family milieu* is included to represent the influence of the social environment and family context on obesity-related health risk. Second, the 5As *(Ask, Assess, Advise, Agree, Assist)* of Obesity Management for adults were developed for clinicians working in primary care to help to promote clinician-patient communication, assessments for obesity, and specific planning for follow-up care [18]. Preliminary evidence suggests that this tool helps clinicians to initiate obesity management and increases the likelihood of follow-up care [19]. A family-centered adaptation of the 5As has been developed for pediatric practice. Finally, since rapport and collaboration are highly valued by clinicians and families alike [5] and since positive, family-centered interactions enhance collaboration and reduce attrition [20], researchers developed a tool for clinicians called CONversation Cards®. The cards include approximately 40 individual statements common to families trying to make and maintain healthy lifestyle changes (e.g., 'I like it when my doctor explains medical terms to me'). Pilot testing showed that (i) the cards can be easily incorporated into day-to-day clinical practice; (ii) families liked using the cards and found them relevant and easy to understand; and (iii) families selected numerous cards, an observation that highlights the variety of issues that families experience in managing pediatric obesity [21]. The CONversation Cards© as well as the adult and pediatric versions of the 5As of Obesity Management are available online from the Canadian Obesity Network (www.obesitynetwork.ca).

Barriers to Accessing Health Services: Families commonly experience barriers to lifestyle change, including limited financial resources, time lost at work/school, difficulty with time management, and perceived self-efficacy to change lifestyle habits. To help to address some of these barriers and optimize families' participation, strategies have included (i) offering health services during evenings and weekends; (ii) providing financial assistance for parking and public transportation; (iii) sharing relevant information through clinic newsletters; (iv) reminding families by telephone regarding upcoming appointments; (v) encouraging participation in clinical and health services research, which often includes financial incentives or tokens of appreciation; and (vi) establishing peer-group programs for support and accountability. Re-evaluation of challenges experienced at initiation and throughout the treatment process can help families to remove barriers and allows clinicians to tailor care to best meet families' needs.

Many primary care-based clinicians encounter frustration because they lack local services for nutrition counselling and accessible community resources for families. It is not uncommon for families to experience long wait times after referral to pediatric specialists and tertiary weight management programs. While waiting, many families have limited access to appropriate support services. In our experience, the children with obesity who are at greatest health risk are not always given the highest priority for assessment and intervention. As with adults [16], the allocation of resources for managing pediatric obesity could benefit from an improved triaging system to help to ensure that those who require more urgent care or who possess more extensive health risks receive appropriate care in a timely manner.

Conclusion

There are a number of common challenges in managing pediatric obesity, many of which relate to factors beyond intervention efficacy or effectiveness. These challenges demonstrate the urgency to identify, disseminate, and implement evidence-based strategies to prevent pediatric obesity using 'upstream' strategies that are available to families in primary care and public health settings. Future areas of research should focus on increasing the availability and accessibility of effective lifestyle change and weight management services through distance support-based options (e.g., eHealth technologies [22, 23]) that can support families where they live, particularly for those living in rural or remote areas. By working in multidisciplinary teams and employing FCC to approach the specific needs of children and families in pediatric weight management, we can make progress in establishing acceptable and effective health care for children with obesity and their families.

References

1 Committee on Hospital Care Institute for Patient Family-Centered Care: Patient- and family-centered care and the pediatrician's role. Pediatrics 2012;129: 394–404.

2 Epstein LH, Paluch RA, Roemmich JN, Beecher MD: Family-based obesity treatment, then and now: twenty-five years of pediatric obesity treatment. Health Psychol 2007;27:381–391.

3 Puhl RM, Peterson JL, Luedicke J: Parental perceptions of weight terminology that providers use with youth. Pediatrics 2011;128:e786–e793.

4 Lau DC, Douketis JS, Morrison KM, Hramiak IM, Sharma AM, Ur E: 2006 Canadian clinical practice guidelines on the management and prevention of obesity in adults and children. CMAJ 2007;176:s1–s13.

5 Farnesi BC, Newton AS, Holt NL, Sharma AM, Ball GDC: Exploring collaboration between clinicians and parents to optimize pediatric weight management. Patient Educ Couns 2012;87:10–17.

6 Reilly J, Kelly J: Long-term impact of overweight and obesity in childhood and adolescence on morbidity and premature mortality in adulthood: systematic review. Int J Obese 2010;35:891–898.

7 Russell-Mayhew S, McVey G, Bardick A, Ireland A: Mental health, wellness, and childhood overweight/obesity. J Obese 2012;2012:281801.

8 Miller WR: Motivational interviewing: research, practice, and puzzles. Addict Behav 1996;6:835–842.

9 Beck AT: Cognitive therapy: past, present, and future. J Consult Clin Psychol 1993;61:194–198.

10 Puhl RM, Heuer CA: The stigma of obesity: a review and update. Obesity 2009;17:941–964.

11 He M, Piche L, Clarson CL, Callaghan C, Harris BS: Childhood overweight and obesity management: a national perspective of primary health care providers' views, practices, perceived barriers and needs. Paediatr Child Healt 2010;15:419–426.

12 Story MT, Neumark-Stzainer DR, Sherwood NE, Holt K, Sofka D, Trowbridge FL, Barlow SE: Management of child and adolescent obesity: attitudes, barriers, skills, and training needs among health care professionals. Pediatrics 2002;110:210–214.

13 Health Canada: Eating well with Canada's food guide. 2007. www.hc-sc.gc.ca/fn-an/food-guide-aliment/index-eng.php (accessed November 4, 2014).

14 Canadian Society for Exercise Physiology: Canadian physical activity guidelines/Canadian sedentary behaviour guidelines. 2012. www.csep.ca/guidelines (accessed November 4, 2014).

15 De Onis M, Lobstein T: Defining obesity risk status in the general childhood population: which cut-offs should we use? Int J Pediatr Obes 2010;5:458–460.
16 Sharma AM, Kushner RF: A proposed clinical staging system for obesity. Int J Obes 2009;33:289–295.
17 Hadjiyannakis S, Buchholz A, Chanoine JP, Hamilton J, Jetha MM, Birken C, Morrison KM, SHarma AM, Ball GDC: The Edmonton Obesity Staging System for Pediatrics (EOSS-P): a proposed clinical staging system for pediatric obesity. Can J Diabetes 2013;37:s240–s240.
18 Vallis M, Piccinni-Vallis H, Sharma AM, Freedhoff Y: Clinical review: modified 5As: minimal intervention for obesity counseling in primary care. Can Fam Physician 2013;59:27–31.
19 Rueda-Clausen CF, Benterud E, Bond T, Olszowka R, Vallis MT, Sharma AM: Effect of implementing the 5As of obesity management framework on provider-patient interactions in primary care. Clin Obes 2013;4:39–44.
20 Farnesi BC, Ball GDC, Newton AS: Family-health professional relations in pediatric weight management: an integrative review. Pediatr Obes 2012;7: 175–186.
21 Ball GDC, Farnesi BC, Newton AS, Holt NL, Geller J, Sharma AM, Johnson ST, MAtteson CL, Finegood DT: Join the conversation! The development and preliminary application of conversation cards in pediatric weight management. J Nutr Educ Behav 2013; 5:476–478.
22 Nguyen B, Kornman KP, Baur LA: A review of electronic interventions for prevention and treatment of overweight and obesity in young people. Obes Rev 2011;12:e298–e314.
23 Smith AJ, Skow S, Bodurtha J, Sanjay K: Health information technology in screening and treatment of child obesity: a systematic review. Pediatrics 2013; 131:e894–e902.

Dr. Geoff D.C. Ball, Associate Professor
8B, Pediatric Centre for Weight and Health, Edmonton General Continuing Care Centre
Stollery Children's Hospital, Alberta Health Services
11111 Jasper Ave.
Edmonton, AB, T5K 0L4 (Canada)
E-Mail gdball@ualberta.ca

Author Index

Subject Index